Eating
Plant-Based

Scientific answers to your nutrition questions

This book is dedicated to our beloved family and loved ones, who continually inspire and support us. We are so blessed to walk our journey with you.

Eating Plant-Based

Scientific answers to your nutrition questions

Dr Shireen Kassam and Dr Zahra Kassam

Foreword by Kate Strong

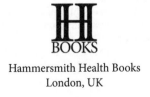

Hammersmith Health Books
London, UK

First published in 2022 by Hammersmith Health Books
– an imprint of Hammersmith Books Limited
4/4A Bloomsbury Square, London WC1A 2RP, UK
www.hammersmithbooks.co.uk

Reprinted 2022

Disclaimer: This book is designed to provide helpful information on the
subjects discussed. It is not meant to be used, nor should it be used, to diagnose
or treat any medical condition. For diagnosis or treatment of any medical
problem, consult your own physician or healthcare provider. The publisher and
authors are not responsible for any specific health or allergy needs that may
require medical supervision and are not liable for any damages or negative
consequences from any treatment, action, application or preparation, to any
person reading or following the information in this book. References are
provided for informational purposes only and do not constitute endorsement of
any websites or other sources. Readers should be aware that the websites listed
in this book may change. The information and references included are up to
date at the time of writing but given that medical evidence progresses, it may
not be up to date at the time of reading.

British Library Cataloguing in Publication Data: A CIP record of this book is
available from the British Library.

Print ISBN 978-1-78161-194-4
Ebook ISBN 978-1-78161-195-1

Commissioning editor: Georgina Bentliff
Designed and typeset by: Julie Bennett of Bespoke Publishing Ltd, UK
Cover design by: Madeline Meckiffe
Cover image: Shutterstock by Craevschii Family
Author image (Shireen Hassam): @iouliakonovalovphotography on Instagram
Index: Dr Laurence Errington
Production: Deborah Wehner of Moatvale Press Ltd, UK
Printed and bound by: TJ Books Ltd, Cornwall, UK

Contents

Contents in detail

Contents in detail

Contents in detail

About the authors

Dr Zahra and Dr Shireen Kassam are sisters and cancer doctors who between them have nearly 40 years of clinical experience in treating patients with cancer on both sides of the Atlantic. In recent years they have developed a shared interest in and appreciation of the power of lifestyle medicine to improve the quality of life and outcomes for their patients. This has culminated in board certification as Lifestyle Medicine Physicians from the International Board of Lifestyle Medicine. They have co-authored a book chapter on food and health in *Rethinking Food and Agriculture: New Ways Forward* and are together editing the forthcoming *Plant-Based Nutrition in Clinical Practice.*

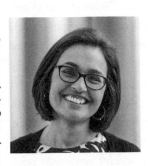

Dr Shireen Kassam MB BS, FRCPATH, PHD, DIPIBLM is a Consultant Haematologist and Honorary Senior Lecturer at King's College Hospital, London with a specialist interest in the treatment of patients with lymphoma (cancer of the lymphatic system). She is also passionate about promoting plant-based nutrition for the prevention and reversal of chronic diseases and for maintaining optimal health after treatment for cancer.

Shireen qualified as a medical doctor in 2000, initially training

@iouliakonovalovphotography on Instagram

xiii

in general medicine, and gaining Membership of the Royal College of Physicians (MRCP) in 2003. She then specialised in Haematology and achieved Fellowship of the Royal College of Pathologists (FRCPath) in 2008. During training, she took time out to undertake a PhD (University of London, 2011). Her research investigated the role of selenium, an essential micronutrient, in sensitising cancer cells to chemotherapy. She was able to show that supra-nutritional doses of selenium could enhance the action of chemotherapy in the laboratory. She has published a number of peer-reviewed papers in the field of lymphoma.

She discovered the power of nutrition for the prevention and treatment of disease in 2013 and since then has been following a whole-food plant-based diet. She has immersed herself in the science of nutrition and health and completed the eCornell certification in plant-based nutrition. In 2019 she became certified as a Lifestyle Medicine Physician by the International Board of Lifestyle Medicine. She is also a certified CHIP (Complete Health Improvement Program) practitioner.

Shireen founded Plant-Based Health Professionals UK in 2018, a community interest company whose mission is to provide evidence-based education and advocacy on plant-based nutrition. Since then, she has been appointed as Visiting Professor of Plant-Based Nutrition at Winchester University where she developed and facilitates the UK's only university-based CPD-accredited course on plant-based nutrition for healthcare professionals. In January 2021, she co-founded and launched the UK's first CQC (Care Quality Commission) registered, online, multi-disciplinary, plant-based lifestyle medicine healthcare service, Plant Based Health Online. She is also a member of the Research Advisory Committee for the Vegan Society. Her work has been published by *The Times, Mail Online, The Mirror, Metro, Vice, Plant Based News* and *BBC Food*. She is an acclaimed national and international speaker and is featured in the 2021 documentary *Eating Our Way to Extinction*.

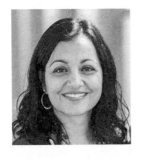

Dr Zahra Kassam MB BS, FRCPC, MSc, DIPABLM is a Radiation Oncologist at the Stronach Regional Cancer Centre in Ontario, Canada, and an Assistant Professor in the Department of Radiation Oncology at the University of Toronto. Zahra received her medical degree from the Imperial College of Science, Technology and Medicine in 1995, completed her specialist training in Clinical Oncology in the UK, followed by three years of clinical and research fellowship training at the Princess Margaret Cancer Centre, Canada, with a Masters in Clinical Epidemiology at the University of Toronto.

Her areas of clinical practice are in gastrointestinal and breast cancers. She has published a number of peer-reviewed papers on these malignancies, as well as in education and mentorship.

A few years ago, Zahra discovered the significant body of evidence demonstrating the benefits of nutrition in the prevention and management of chronic diseases, not taught at any stage of her medical training. She is a certified Lifestyle Medicine Physician with the American Board of Lifestyle Medicine and has completed the eCornell certification in plant-based nutrition and the Plant-Based Nutrition course at the University of Winchester. Zahra co-founded Plant-Based Canada, a non-profit organisation, in 2019, with the goal of educating the public and health professionals on the evidence-based benefits of plant-based whole food nutrition for individual and planetary health. Their inaugural event was held in 2019, the first Canadian Plant-Based Nutrition conference in Toronto.

Acknowledgements

We wish to express our sincere gratitude to all who have made this book possible. Special thanks to Rohini Bajekal, who took the time to read the book and provided invaluable insights; to Kate Strong, for writing the foreword and sharing her inspiring plant-based journey; and of course to Georgina Bentliff, director of Hammersmith Health Books, for her support, expertise, care and realisation of this book.

Our deep love and gratitude go to our beloved family and loved ones for their constant support and inspiration.

Foreword

Even after being World Triathlon Champion in long-distance triathlon and breaking three world records in static cycling, covering 433.09 miles in 24 hours, I still get asked, 'Where do you get your protein?' I wonder if meat-eating athletes get asked the same because, isn't protein required for every person?

I do appreciate why I'm asked this question, and typically it's because we, as a society, rarely question what we are told and presented as 'facts', such as meat being the best source of protein, an essential macronutrient for a balanced diet.

Growing up, I believed my mother and teachers at school when they said that eating a little bit of everything was a balanced diet. I didn't question the validity of this statement, nor explore the moral or ethical aspects of what was on my plate at dinner time. It was not until I went through a personal trauma that I started to see my actions, and what I ate, from a different angle.

In 2012, my partner of nine years left me just six days before our wedding. On the one hand, I was immensely relieved because, over time, our relationship had deteriorated from a supportive environment into a controlling and toxic place for me. My phone was tracked and I was unable to move freely without his permission, friends were squeezed out of my life and I was afraid to say 'No' to him and express my opinions for fear of his reaction. Yet, on the other hand, I felt overwhelmed. Living alone in Australia, trying to run a hospitality business single-handed and also manage the debt he had left me with after his departure seemed too big for me to manage. I turned to alcohol to help me suppress the anxiety building up in me and also to give me courage to keep moving through the days and numbing the lonesome nights.

After four months of drinking almost every day, I noticed that I was still holding onto the resentment of my ex leaving me to manage the chaos alone. I could see the bitterness on my face when I looked in the mirror and hear it cutting through my words. It was then that I realised I had a choice: I could either allow this past event to define me forever, or I could use it as fuel to create something positive in my life. I chose the latter.

You may be asking how this part of my journey is relevant to a book advocating a plant-based diet yet, for me, they are one and the same. The moment I committed to being responsible for my present frame of mind, I chose to open my eyes to how I interact with the world and the impact I was having within it.

It was around this time that I decided to reignite an old goal of mine. Nine years prior, when I had started dating my ex, I had set the goal of entering an Ironman triathlon – a gruelling 2.4-mile swim and a 112-mile cycle followed by a 26.2-mile marathon run. After finishing a half Ironman, I listened to my ex and decided not to enter the full Ironman, his words of 'You've done enough' holding me back from following my dream. Almost a decade later, the desire to compete in triathlon was reignited and I decided not to cap my potential, setting myself the ambitious target of qualifying for, and winning, world championships.

Being an asthmatic, I struggled with breathing once my runs started reaching 10 kilometres; I couldn't get enough air in. No matter how often I trained, as soon as the distance slipped into double digits I could feel my lungs contracting and I was typically left wheezing and feeling as if I was slowly suffocating.

After a few particularly frustrating runs, a local artisan at the village market suggested that it was the amount of cheese and milk I was consuming that was impacting my running. Initially, my response was disbelief; how could the problem be what I ate, especially dairy – something I'd been told since birth was essential for healthy bones? Desperate to improve, I decided to trial this seemingly ludicrous suggestion and stopped eating any dairy for 30 days. Prior to stopping, I timed myself over a 5-kilometre circuit and my intention was to re-run the same circuit one month later and compare the results.

As it turned out, I didn't need to wait for more than a week before I started noticing the difference. Even within this short time-period, I saw a spike in my speed, running a full 5 seconds per kilometre faster. I also felt better after finishing a run, wheezing a lot less and feeling refreshed rather than exhausted. Even some locals who I ran with occasionally remarked on how much quieter I was, as they were used to hearing me wheeze and chuff before they could see me on our trail runs.

That week had a profound impact on me. It was as if a light bulb had turned on and I could see the link between what I was eating and my performance – something that seems so obvious now, and yet I had ignored or missed up until that point. I knew I could not return to eating dairy after experiencing first-hand how it was triggering my asthma.

Over time, I also noticed more subtle changes from removing dairy from my diet. My skin felt more supple, with fewer areas of intense dryness and less frequent and less extreme break-outs of spots. My hairdresser asked what conditioner I had switched to (I didn't use any conditioner) because my hair was thicker, where it should have been more damaged due to all the swimming in chlorinated swimming pools. Even my father asked whether I was wearing contact lenses because my eyes seemed bluer and brighter than before.

Nothing had changed except for me removing dairy from what I ate and drank.

It was during this period that I started to explore all the food types that I was eating, and the impact they were having on my performance and health. If dairy – something that I had been led to believe by so-called 'experts' was healthy – actually created dis-ease within me, what else was I eating that was actually harming my health?

Next to go was red meat when I realised that, whenever I ate a meat-heavy meal, my recovery time after training was longer than if I ate a plant-heavy meal. Before long, I was eating exclusively whole food and plant-based fuel.

Coming from an engineering background, I wanted to know whether what I was experiencing was an isolated case, or if more people experienced adverse effects while eating animal-based foods. Delving into many Google Scholar searches, there was a lot of noise and conflicting evidence about the benefits versus the drawbacks of eating meat and dairy. Yet, there was one constant. Whenever an article or scientific report boasted about the benefits of eating meat, or negated the link between dairy and asthma, they always appeared to be funded by a dairy or farmers' union. These reports couldn't be unbiased when their primary funder was so linked to the outcomes of promoting eating more meat and dairy.

Today, thankfully, we have researchers and doctors such as Shireen and Zahra Kassam, who are sharing the unbiased truth about the health benefits of switching from meat and dairy to a more natural and plant-based food source. And, thanks to researchers, we are also discovering that there are more than just health benefits to be had from eating more plants and fewer animal-based products. The environmental footprint of having meat and cheese on our plates is significantly larger than purely plants. Soyabeans are being grown in sensitive and much needed areas of our world to feed farmed animals. It is estimated that over 80% of all soyabeans produced are fed to cattle – beans that we humans could thrive on yet choose to feed to cows in order to have our Sunday roast. We are quite literally destroying the habitats that help keep us alive.

And our impact doesn't just reside on the land. Fish numbers are dropping to dangerous levels and algae blooms, which suffocate many miles of ocean, are becoming more frequent, yet we still deny that our actions are having a detrimental, if not devastating, effect on the world.

Over 97% of scientists agree that human activity – with our hunger for meat, for excessive travel and for other irresponsible activities – is impacting the world to an almost irreparable extent. Let us assume that those 97% of scientists are wrong, and the 3% are right who emphatically state that the increase in extreme temperatures, bush fires and flooding is a natural rhythm of this planet? Even so, by turning towards a more nature-conscious way of living and eating more plants, we can only impact the world positively. There is no flip-side to our choosing to be more intentional with our actions and food choices.

Whether we are seeking a means to maintain optimal health, recover from a disease, or reduce our carbon footprint and help combat climate change, assessing and changing what we eat does have a profound and positive impact in all cases. With organisations like Plant-Based Health Professionals UK and Plant-Based Canada popping up across the globe, we can all be supported along the transition from unconscious eating and existing into living a thriving life. We don't have to be one sneeze away from a cold, or live in fear of suffering a heart-attack; we have power and we have a choice. Every one of the five big killers in the UK (heart disease, stroke, cancer, lung disease and liver disease) is directly linked to what we eat, and we can reduce our risk, purely by reducing or removing animal-based products from our diet.

Being able to thrive and have optimal performance isn't reserved for the extreme athlete; it is for each and every one of us, and we can achieve this through awareness, understanding and action. I use my sport as a means to raise awareness and interest in how we can thrive while also supporting the environment we live in, and Shireen and Zahra Kassam are doing similarly with this book. This comprehensive book provides the answers to the common plant-based nutrition questions, backed by the most up-to-date scientific evidence. It will give you the background to help you transition to plant-based eating, deepen your knowledge and give you the confidence to advocate with your friends, family and beyond. I implore you to read this book as if your health, and life, depended on it. In many ways, it holds the key to supporting us all in living a truly healthy life and also ensuring that we leave a world that is as diverse and as beautiful as possible for the generations to come.

Kate Strong
World Champion Triathlete, Engineer, Plant-based Adventurer,
Coach and Consultant, Entrepreneur, Reiki Master,
Philanphropist and 3 x Cycle World Record Holder
https://katestrong.global/

Introduction

This book is for those of you who would like a deeper understanding of the scientific evidence supporting a plant-based diet and its impact on human health. It is for those of you who are already following a plant-based diet and for those who would like to switch to this way of eating but are being put off by family and friends who question your choice and fill your head with doubt. Is it safe to raise children on a plant-based diet? How do you get enough protein? What about calcium? And iodine? The answers to all these questions are simple and straightforward and this book provides the scientific background to our understanding of plant-based diets.

If you are thinking about making the transition, this book will give you the confidence to do so. If you are already following a plant-based diet, it will help you with advocating for and discussing your choice with others in an impartial, evidence-based way. The questions are based around our own experience of advocating and educating family, health professionals, patients and the public on plant-based diets for the last decade.

Chapter 1

Eating plant-based

1.1 Why should I go plant-based?

The decision to adopt a plant-based diet mainly comes down to three broad reasons: concerns for personal health, planetary health and animal justice. It is a loose term without a precise definition, but it signifies the move to a diet centred predominantly around whole plant foods, whilst minimising the consumption of meat, dairy and eggs. In our view, a diet that is more than 85% centred on whole plant foods comes under the term 'plant-based'.

The science supporting plant-based diets for all the reasons mentioned is irrefutable. International reports estimate that a global shift to a plant-based diet could prevent one in five deaths – that is, 11 million lives saved per year – from diet-related illness[1]. One of the most comprehensive analyses of the global farming system, assessing all aspects of the food chain 'from farm to fork', concluded that shifting to a plant-based diet would have a greater impact on planetary health than any other driver of climate change[2]. The benefit for almost 80 billion land animals and two trillion fish killed every year for food is self-evident.

This book focuses on the health aspects of a 100% plant-based diet. The evidence supporting a plant-based diet for maintaining optimal health is now undeniable. Decades of research have confirmed that a plant-based diet can significantly reduce the risk of some of our commonest chronic diseases. A plant-based diet can reduce the risk of heart disease by at least 25%[3, 4, 5], type 2 diabetes by up to 50%[6, 7, 8] and hypertension (high blood pressure) by 60%[9], and can help maintain healthy blood cholesterol levels[10]. Not only that, but a plant-based diet is an effective treatment for many of these same chronic conditions. It is as effective as medication for the treatment of high blood pressure[11] and cholesterol[12,13]. It can be used to effectively treat type 2 diabetes and in many cases even achieve a remission[14, 15, 16]. A plant-based diet, with or without other healthy lifestyle habits, has been shown to arrest the progression of coronary heart disease, with shrinkage of atherosclerotic plaque in the arteries in some patients[17, 18, 19]. As if that were not enough, a plant-based diet has been shown to halt the progression of early stages of prostate cancer in men[20].

These are phenomenal statements to be able to make about a diet. Suffice it to say that even Bill Clinton, former US President, sought out the expertise of one of the founding fathers of the therapeutic use of a plant-based diet, Dr Dean Ornish, after his quadruple heart bypass, and went on to adopt a plant-based diet[21]. This same Ornish Program for Reversing Heart Disease has been paid for by Medicare since 2010, the federal health insurance program in the US, based on the strength of evidence presented showing its ability to halt the progression of coronary heart disease and reduce the need for coronary artery bypass surgery or other similar intervention[22].

There is no doubt remaining for us that a plant-based diet is one of the healthiest choices we can make.

1.2 What is the difference between plant-based and vegan?

Plant-based essentially refers to a diet choice whereas veganism is a social justice movement encompassing justice for non-human animals and humans alike. The term 'vegan' tells you what a person is *not* consuming: meat, eggs, dairy, honey plus any food that would require animals or animal parts in its production. In fact, vegans aim to avoid the use of animals in all aspects of their lives. The term 'vegan diet', however, does not describe what a person is eating, which could be anything from whole plant foods to crisps, chocolates, cakes and other ultra-processed foods. The term 'plant-based' usually refers to a diet-pattern that focuses on whole plant foods. More accurately, it should be referred to as a 'whole-food plant-based (WFPB) diet', which is the term for a healthy vegan diet. This reflects a diet pattern centred around fruit, vegetables, whole grains, legumes (we will come back to these later), nuts and seeds. Ideally, a healthy plant-based diet should minimise added oil, salt and sugar.

1.3 What are some of the commonly used terms?

Vegetarian: a general term for a diet pattern that excludes meat, poultry and fish.

Lacto-ovo vegetarian: a diet that permits the consumption of dairy and eggs.

Lacto-vegetarianism: a diet that permits the consumption of dairy but not eggs.

Pesco-vegetarianism (a term used less frequently): a diet that incorporates seafood in an otherwise vegetarian dietary pattern.

Vegan: a diet that excludes all animal-derived foods, including eggs, dairy and honey.

Flexitarian or 'casual vegetarian': an increasingly popular term used to describe those actively reducing their consumption of meat and dairy, usually to reduce the environmental impact of their diet, but still consuming small amounts of meat, poultry, eggs and dairy.

Plant-based: a dietary pattern that is predominately, but not exclusively comprised of plant foods. Although there is no consensus definition, plant-based diets typically include 85-90% plant-derived foods. In the scientific literature, the term plant-based often incorporates all the terms listed above but predominantly vegan and vegetarian dietary patterns.

Whole-food plant-based diet: a healthy vegan diet composed of fruit, vegetables, whole grains, legumes, nuts and seeds and minimising/avoiding the consumption of added fat, salt and sugar.

1.4 What sort of studies have helped us understand the health benefits of plant-based eating?

Nutrition science is complex and no one study will provide all the answers. In general, a combination of studies is needed to truly understand the impact of diet on health outcomes. Much of our understanding of plant-based diets comes from prospective cohort studies. These are studies in which thousands of participants, who are healthy at the point of recruitment, are followed over the subsequent years and decades. Dietary information is collected at baseline and usually at regular intervals during follow up and this information is correlated with health outcomes, such as the development of heart disease or cancer. There are two large prospective cohort studies that have informed us about the health of vegetarians and vegans. The Adventist Health Study-2 (AHS-2) includes 96,000 Adventists from North America and started recruitment in 2001. The EPIC-Oxford study includes 65,000 participants from the UK and started recruitment in 1993. Both studies are ongoing and include around a third of participants who are vegetarian or vegan. There are other smaller studies investigating the health of vegetarians and vegans that will be referred to in this book, including the Tzu Chi Health Study involving Buddhists from Taiwan[23].

Many important prospective cohort studies, such as the Nurses' Health Study and the Health Professionals Follow-up Study (HPFS) conducted from Harvard University, do not include large numbers of vegetarians and vegans. To study the impact of eating whole plant-foods, researchers have developed the plant-based diet index (PBDI) which scores foods either positively or negatively and correlates the consumption of these foods with health outcomes. In the PBDI, all animal-derived foods and unhealthy plant foods, such as refined grains, sugar-sweetened beverages, sweets and desserts, are given a negative score and healthy whole plant foods are given a positive score[5]. The dietary information from study participants is scored accordingly and then correlated with health outcomes. When researchers have used the PBDI to analyse dietary data from large cohort studies, they have found that participants who consumed the healthiest plant foods and the least animal-derived and processed foods had a significantly lower risk of certain chronic conditions. Examples include a 25% reduction in the risk of coronary heart disease[24], 15% reduction in the risk of cancer[25], 24% reduction in the risk of fatty liver[26], 34% reduction in the risk of type 2 diabetes[27], 14% reduction in the risk of developing kidney failure[28], 10% reduction in the risk of stroke and even a 10% reduction in the risk of early death[29]. However, it's worth noting that most studies have found that those consuming an unhealthy plant-based diet when compared with omnivores do not receive health benefits and in fact may increase the risk of certain chronic conditions.

The main criticism of these types of observational study is that they demonstrate association and not causation. However, it was just these types of study that showed that tobacco smoking caused cancer and that trans-fat consumption increased the risk of cardiovascular disease[30]. If such studies are conducted in a robust manner, they can provide important information on diet and health.

Prospective cohort studies are complemented by the findings of studies that investigate mechanisms by which certain foods impact our health. For example, studies have shown that consumption of animal foods increases the level of the growth hormone IGF-1 (insulin-like growth factor 1) in the blood. Elevated IGF-1 levels are associated with an increased risk of various cancers and in the laboratory IGF-1 increases the growth of cancer cells. The combination of these types of data gives us a plausible explanation for the finding that vegans have a significantly lower incidence of cancer[31, 32].

The ideal study is considered to be a randomised controlled trial (RCT) of one diet pattern versus another, whilst ensuring all other lifestyle variables, such as physical activity and alcohol consumption, remain constant. These types of study are notoriously difficult to conduct. Not only are they hugely expensive, but it is also often nigh on impossible to ensure study participants adhere to the prescribed diet over long time periods unless the food is provided for them, and often for their family members too, which clearly is not practical on a large scale. People's lifestyles are highly variable and don't necessarily remain constant over time. So often these RCTs are conducted on a small scale for short time periods. Nonetheless, when they are well designed and rigorously conducted, they provide invaluable information that can help support the findings of observational studies.

In some instances, it is unethical to conduct a randomised study. For example, the strength of evidence connecting smoking and cancer is such that conducting a RCT in which half of the participants were required to smoke and the other not would be considered unethical in anyone's book.

When there are enough studies on a particular topic, the results can be brought together and combined in a systematic review or meta-analysis. These types of study are often considered the best available evidence[33]. However, they are not without issues as the validity of the results are dependent on what data are used in the analysis and how the analysis is conducted.

The most robust type of systematic review is often considered to be those conducted by Cochrane, a British charitable organisation bringing together thousands of volunteer experts from around the world to analyse and synthesise the results of studies on healthcare interventions. However, even Cochrane has come under criticism lately due to its relationship with the pharmaceutical industry[34].

Given the limitations of RCTs, and that current approaches to assessing the strength of evidence rely heavily on RCTs, a new construct called 'hierarchies of evidence applied to lifestyle medicine' (HEALM) has been developed to assess the strength of evidence relevant to the impact of nutrition and other lifestyle behaviours on health outcomes. HEALM incorporates the variety of sources of evidence available and synthesises their contributions into one rating[35, 36]. Interestingly, a Cochrane systematic review in 2014 concluded that RCTs and observational studies tend to produce similar effect sizes for a range of health outcomes and that disagreements in study conclusions are likely due to other study characteristics, such as testing different hypotheses or duration of follow-up rather than the study design alone[37].

1.5 Aren't humans designed to eat meat and dairy?

Humans are omnivores. We have a choice. We can choose to include meat, dairy and eggs in our diet, but these foods are not essential. There are no nutrients within animal-derived food that cannot be obtained from whole plant foods (the one exception being vitamin B12, see section 10.3). In fact, the opposite is true. Without sufficient plant foods, human health and well-being suffer. Plant foods are essential for vitamins and minerals such as vitamins C, E, K and folate, and of course fibre.

Humans for most of history have been gatherers rather than

hunters. Nutritional anthropologists have estimated that the nutrient intake of prehistoric humans included as much as 100 grams of fibre per day[38]. That's a lot of plant foods! Hunting animals for food is challenging for humans and our anatomy and physiology are in fact more adapted to eating plants. Just look at your canine teeth, for example. They are short and blunt, unlike animals that rely on meat like lions, whose canines are long, sharp and curved. Our canines would not be very effective at stabbing, tearing and killing prey.

The majority of the world's population does not have the ability to digest lactose, the main sugar in dairy, beyond weaning[39]. This is because the enzyme lactase does not persist in mammals once a mothers' milk is unnecessary in the diet. Without the production of lactase in the gut, the consumption of dairy can lead to unpleasant symptoms such as nausea, diarrhoea and bloating. This is termed 'lactose intolerance'. Lactose intolerance ranges from up to 30% in Caucasian populations to up to 90% in Asian, Indian and African populations and, overall, this is the norm in 70% of the global population. The adaptation for digesting lactose, lactase persistence, arose around 5000-10,000 years ago, mainly in European populations in line with domestication of cows and the production of dairy[40]. An evolutionary advantage for this adaptation does not seem to be apparent. It is worth mentioning that no other species drinks milk beyond a young age, their own mother's, or the milk of another species.

Some of the healthiest and longest-lived populations on this planet, found in regions of the World termed 'Blue Zones', have in common a diet that is at least 85% plant-based, with some, such as vegans in Loma Linda, California, consuming no animal foods at all[41].

Regardless of our adaptations and ability to consume meat, dairy and eggs, the question we should be asking is 'do we need to?' The answer is a resounding NO.

1.6 My doctor told me I had to eat meat?

What you have to understand about doctors in general, is that they will have received very little or no nutrition education during medical school[42, 43]. Historically, our nutrition education at best amounted to a few hours of teaching within a course that overall lasts 5–6 years, with an emphasis on nutritional biochemistry and deficiencies rather than the clinical application of nutrition. By the time we qualify, our brains have been filled with the latest guideline on the management of various clinical conditions that predominantly focus on medications, procedures or medical interventions.

The initial training for all doctors involves treating established chronic illness, be it on the acute medical or surgical wards or in the emergency department. The impact of nutrition and lifestyle factors for promoting health and well-being is soon forgotten as we firefight our way through the first few years hoping we don't make an error, trying to keep up to date with new information whilst attempting to pass postgraduate exams. For most doctors, their personal health and well-being deteriorate as they try to juggle the demands of work with their personal and family lives[44].

So, the nutrition advice you may receive from most doctors will not necessarily be based on the latest evidence but will most likely reflect the preferences and biases of the doctor. Studies show that doctors who undertake regular physical activity, for example, are much more likely to promote the benefits of physical activity to their patients[45]. In the same way, a doctor who continues to eat red and processed meat is likely to tell their patients that eating these foods in moderation is fine and that meat is necessary in the diet.

As doctors following a plant-based diet ourselves, we are much more likely to spend time explaining why limiting and ideally avoiding red and processed meat in the diet is the best option. Luckily, medical education is changing and more nutrition and lifestyle training is being incorporated into the medical school curricula and postgraduate education, driven by demands from medical students, doctors and health professional organisations[46, 47]. There will be an inevitable lag between implementing this education and the time when all doctors will be able to provide evidence-based nutrition counselling to their patients. New knowledge can take a long time to become established into clinical practice, oftentimes over a decade[48]. Behavioural changes also take time. For example, it took more than 40 years from the first Surgeon General's report on smoking and cancer in 1964 for the UK to ban smoking inside hospital buildings in 2007 and even longer to ban smoking anywhere on the premises. We have a way to go before processed meat is banned from hospital canteens and food outlets since its classification as a group 1 carcinogen by the WHO (World Health Organization) in 2015.

Our advice: make sure you do your own research and acknowledge the limitations of your doctor who will be super-specialised in their own area but cannot be an expert in everything. Find a doctor, dietitian or nutritionist who is trained in nutrition and, in particular, plant-based nutrition.

1.7 Do you have to be 100% plant-based to derive health benefits?

The healthiest diet patterns are those that are predominantly plant-based but not necessarily 100%. The diet of the Blue Zones, five regions of the world where people live the longest, healthiest lives, is at least 85% plant-based with consumption of beans featuring highly in all these regions. Meat is eaten infrequently, maybe five times a month and for special occasions[41].

The Eat-Lancet commission brought together 37 scientists from 16 countries to come up with a diet pattern that would not only sustain human health but sustain planetary health for a population of 10 billion people by 2050[49]. It came up with the

Planetary Health Plate, an eating pattern in which only 13% of calories are derived from animal foods, with the vast majority of calories and nutrients obtained from plant sources. If this diet pattern was adopted globally, the report predicts that 11 million lives could be saved from diet-related illness every year. The report is clear that animal foods are not required in the diet and, if consumed, should be minimised. Their only exception to this was the recommendation on fish consumption that will be discussed later (Chapter 5).

Nonetheless, let's be clear. It is absolutely possible to maintain optimal health and wellbeing on a 100% plant-based or healthy vegan diet. This is supported by most of the major national and international dietetic and nutrition organisations around the world[50]. So then, it once again comes down to a choice as to whether you decide to be 100% plant-based or 87% plant-based. For those who are equally or more concerned about environmental and animal justice issues relating to our food choices, rest assured you will not be compromising your personal health by adopting a 100% plant-based diet.

1.8 Are there benefits for weight management?

Overweight and obesity are now at epidemic proportions around the world and a major factor in the rise of non-communicable diseases, including cardiovascular disease, certain cancers, type 2 diabetes, chronic kidney disease and dementia[51]. Our diet choices are the main determinant of body weight, and a diet centred around whole plant foods is the best way to maintain a healthy weight. There are a number of reasons for this:

- Plant foods are naturally low in calories yet high in nutrients. On a plant-based diet you therefore eat fewer calories without having to overly restrict portion size[52, 53, 54], with the high fibre intake contributing to a greater feeling of fullness despite an overall lower calorie intake.

- The naturally lower fat content of a plant-based diet results in greater loss of body fat when weight loss is required[55].

- There is greater loss of energy or calories after consuming a plant-based meal – post-prandial energy expenditure – than after consuming one that includes meat[54]. (Post prandial metabolism and the thermic effect of food is a natural physiologic process in the body, accounting for 10% of all energy expenditure.)

- Plant foods also better regulate the appetite hormones produced in our gut and brain, helping us to feel more satiated[55, 56].

In observational studies of vegan health, participants consuming a vegan diet have been much more likely to maintain a healthy weight than those consuming animal foods[7, 57]. Over time, those eating the most fruit, vegetables, whole grains and beans are most likely to prevent weight gain compared to those consuming more animal and processed foods[58, 59]. Randomised studies have also confirmed the benefits of a healthy plant-based diet for weight loss[60, 61]. The BROAD study was a RCT using a low-fat WFPB diet in a community setting for obesity, ischaemic heart disease or diabetes[62]. The intervention group was not required to restrict calories or undertake physical activity and was compared with a control group that continued their usual care. Patients were followed up to 12 months. The intervention led to a significant and sustained reduction in weight and body mass index (BMI) at all time points when compared with the control group. This is notable, as it was a community intervention such that what people ate was not controlled in any way other than through upfront dietary education. The authors concluded that this study 'achieved greater weight loss at 6 and 12 months than any other trial that does not limit energy intake or mandate regular exercise'. A WFPB diet has also been shown to be better at reducing fat inside the muscle and liver cells and thus reversing insulin resistance[54]. The more plant-based foods in the diet the better the health of the gut microbiome, an important factor in maintaining a healthy body weight[63].

All in all, the evidence stacks up in favour of a plant-based diet for maintaining a healthy body weight and has been shown to be a sustainable long-term solution for preventing weight gain.

1.9 What about the Mediterranean diet? Isn't that a healthy way of eating?

Yes, this is correct. The Mediterranean diet is a healthy diet pattern, which is why for four years in a row it has been voted the 'best diet overall' by a panel of experts for the *US World and News Report* on best diets (2021). There are, however, a few things to consider before concluding whether the Mediterranean diet is better than a 100% plant-based diet.

The Mediterranean diet is not simply a single diet because the Mediterranean region is large, with a variety of traditional ways of eating. The usual image that comes to mind when thinking about the Mediterranean diet is sitting on a white, sandy beach on a warm summer's day sipping red wine and eating olives and maybe even grilling fish on an open barbeque. In fact, Sardinia in Italy and Ikaria in Greece are both Blue Zones, regions of the world where people live the longest and healthiest lives and have the greatest chance of living to 100 years old. But what is it about the Mediterranean diet that makes it so healthy? Well it turns about that researchers have asked just this question[64].

What they found when analysing dietary data from more than 20,000 men and women from Greece was that the components of the diet that were associated with the greatest health benefits were the vegetables, legumes, nuts, fruit and unsaturated fatty acids (from plant sources). The foods that did not appear to impact health outcomes in the Mediterranean diet were dairy, fish and meat. So, the diet is healthy *because* of the strong emphasis on plant-based foods and *not because* of the animal-based foods that are included.

The PREDIMED study is always cited as the one that proves how good the Mediterranean diet is for cardiovascular health[65]. This study assigned 7447 participants who were at high risk of developing cardiovascular disease (CVD) to three groups – two intervention groups and a control group. The intervention groups were assigned to a Mediterranean diet with either added olive oil (50 grams/4 tablespoons) or a daily portion of nuts (30 grams). The control group were asked to follow a low-fat diet pattern, but it should be noted they did not achieve the planned lowering of fat. After following the participants for 4.8 years, the results showed only minimal weight loss in each group, with no difference between the intervention and control groups. The main difference in outcome was in a combined reduction in the chance of suffering a heart attack or stroke or dying from CVD. The main contributor to this significant finding was a 40% reduction in the risk of stroke in the nut-consuming group rather than any reduction in heart attacks or risk of dying from CVD or, indeed, any cause.

In contrast, when the PREDIMED study was analysed using the plant-based diet index (see section 1.4 for more information on this index) there was a significant reduction in the risk of all-cause *and* cardiovascular mortality in those consuming a diet with a high plant-based diet score, suggesting once again that the whole plant foods in the Mediterranean diet are those conferring the benefit[66]. The authors of this analysis concluded: 'we provide evidence to support that the simple advice to increase the consumption of plant-derived foods with compensatory reductions in the consumption of foods from animal sources confers a survival advantage to older subjects at high cardiovascular risk.'

There are very few direct, head-to-head comparisons of the Mediterranean diet with a 100% plant-based diet. There has been one of a Mediterranean diet compared with a vegetarian diet[67]. The CARDIVEG study randomly assigned 118 overweight participants with high blood lipids or glucose, but who were not on any medication, to either one of the two diet patterns. It was a three-month intervention with both diet groups having the same but reduced calorie intake. After the three months both groups crossed over to the other diet pattern. It was found that both diets were equally effective in reducing body weight, body mass index and fat mass, with no significant differences between them. However, the vegetarian diet was more effective in reducing total cholesterol, low-density lipoprotein (LDL) cholesterol and insulin levels, whereas the Mediterranean diet led to a greater reduction in triglyceride levels.

In another very small study comparing the vegan diet with the Mediterranean diet for cardiovascular health in 24 young, healthy volunteers, the Mediterranean diet led to improvements in microvascular function and the vegan diet led to a greater reduction in total cholesterol and weight[69]. It is worth noting that the vegan diet in this study was relatively high in fat, with participants consuming 35% of calories from fat.

At the start of 2021, the long anticipated results of a head-to-head comparison of the Mediterranean diet with a low-fat WFPB diet were published[53]. A low-fat WFPB diet is a healthy version of a vegan diet, which in clinical studies has been shown to have excellent effects on health outcomes. Prior research had shown that a low-fat WFPB diet (meaning avoidance of added processed oils and high-fat plant foods such as nuts) had the ability to halt the progression of atherosclerosis and in some cases even shown regression of atherosclerotic plaques[18, 19, 69].

So, how was this trial conducted and what did it show? The study randomly assigned 62 overweight adults to either a Mediterranean or a low-fat vegan diet for 16 weeks. After a four-week 'washout' period in which participants returned to their baseline diet, they then crossed over to the alternative diet for a further 16 weeks. Both groups could eat as much as they wanted. The Mediterranean diet followed the diet in the PREDIMED study, described above, and included 50 grams of olive oil daily. The vegan diet was intended to contain approximately 75% carbohydrates, 15% protein and 10% fat from whole-plant sources, no added oil and a B12 supplement. Body weight, blood pressure, body composition, insulin resistance and glucose tolerance were measured before and after each phase.

What were the results? The actual fat intake was 43% of calories in the Mediterranean group and 17% in the vegan group. Although participants could eat as much as they wanted, the vegan group consumed around 500 fewer calories per day and had a higher intake of fibre and lower intakes of saturated fat and cholesterol. The vegan group lost an average of 6 kilograms, but the Mediterranean-diet group lost no weight. The vegan group also had significant reductions in body fat and visceral fat and significant improvements in blood total and LDL-cholesterol levels and insulin sensitivity. These parameters did not change in the Mediterranean diet group. Both groups had reductions in blood pressure but there was a greater effect in the Mediterranean diet group.

All in all, the healthy vegan diet held its own against the Mediterranean diet, and in some areas outperformed it. The authors hypothesised that the greater reduction in blood pressure in the Mediterranean diet group might have been due to the high content of monounsaturated fat and vitamin E, and the antioxidant function of olive oil. We wonder how the vegan diet would have fared with a daily tablespoon of flaxseeds or portion of nuts added (see Chapter 9). Nonetheless, these results go some way to explaining why the Ornish low-fat WFPB diet has been voted the top heart-healthy diet for 10 years in a row by the *US World and News Report*.

Researchers have tried to improve upon the traditional Mediterranean diet by adding more plant foods, green tea, walnuts and Mankai (duckweed, discussed in section 10.3), and including less meat, the so-called 'Green Mediterranean diet'. No surprise – studies showed that this 'greener' version outperformed the standard version[70, 71].

Our conclusion is that the Mediterranean diet is beneficial *because* of the emphasis on whole plant foods. The other components, such as fish, poultry, alcohol and dairy for example, act to make this diet more acceptable within our cultural and societal norms but are not essential components of the diet for health. It is, however, certainly very much better than the typical Western-style diet pattern.

1.10 Isn't a plant-based diet too high in carbs?

We sometimes need to be reminded that carbohydrates, or 'carbs' for short, are not a food group. Carbohydrates are found in all plant foods. To therefore conclude that carbohydrates are all bad is an oversimplification that has led to a lot of confusion. Carbohydrates are found in the healthiest foods on this planet: fruit, vegetables, whole grains and beans. The reason carbs are given a bad name is because all carbohydrates are eventually digested by the body into sugar or glucose, which is used for energy or stored as glycogen. Consuming sugar in excess of calorie requirements is bad for health and therefore the erroneous conclusion reached by some is that all carbohydrates must be bad. The types of carbs that are not healthy are from foods that have been refined and thus have lost many of their beneficial nutrients, such as fibre, vitamins and minerals. These include table sugar and white flour products, such as bread, cakes, pastries and even white rice. They also include the free sugar in sugar-sweetened beverages and the high fructose corn syrup used in sauces and other processed foods. Free sugar, in all its many forms, and refined carbohydrates are often found in unhealthy foods that are also high in fat, such as donuts and ice-cream. Sticking to whole food sources of carbs, such as whole grain bread, brown rice, quinoa, beans, fruit and vegetables, is absolutely the best thing for health, and the high consumption of healthy carbs is of no concern on a plant-based diet.

The optimal amount of carbohydrates continues to be a topic of debate and often detracts from the simple message of eating more healthy plant foods. If you consider the traditional diet of people from Okinawa in Japan, another Blue Zone, 85% of their energy intake comes from carbohydrates, with sweet potato being the main staple food, then we cannot possibly conclude that carbohydrates are bad[73]. It may be perfectly possible to eat a lower-carb plant-based diet by increasing the consumption of plant-based protein and fat from olives, nuts and avocados. The Eco-Atkins diet designed by Dr David Jenkins and researchers at the University of Toronto is such a low-carb plant-based diet and may have some advantages for cardio-metabolic health[74]. However, most people following a low-carb diet for the short-term benefits of weight loss and glucose control are usually replacing healthy carbs with meat (which is devoid of carbs) and other animal-sources of protein and fat. We know from a number of population studies that a low-carb diet high in animal foods results in an increased risk of cardiovascular disease, cancer and early death in the longer term[74, 75]. What is often forgotten is that when carbohydrates and glycogen stores are in short supply, protein can be converted to glucose and this occurs in preference to using fat stores and thus low-carb diets can result in loss of lean muscle mass[77]. In addition, protein also stimulates the release of insulin, so the theory that high-protein diets that are low in sugar do not stress the pancreas is also misguided[78].

A plant-based diet has been tested head-to-head with a low-carb animal-based diet in a type of study called a metabolic ward study[52]. This is a rigorous study in which participants are admitted to a clinical facility, all the food is provided, and they are intensively monitored and investigated. For this study, participants could eat as much as they wanted. On the plant-based diet, participants consumed significantly fewer calories. Both diets led to improvements in fasting glucose and insulin levels, but the plant-based diet resulted in greater weight and body fat loss and improvements in cholesterol levels. The low-carb group lost mainly water weight and muscle mass, developed a degree of insulin resistance and a rise in LDL-cholesterol levels. The low-carb diet did improve triglyceride levels, which worsened on the plant-based diet.

All in all, there are no robust data to support a low-carb approach for long-term health or any adverse effects of a high-carb plant-based diet. In fact, an animal-based low-carb diet will adversely impact long-term health.

1.11 Isn't it sugar that is the problem, not animal foods?

There are many components of a typical Western-style diet that are unhealthy, and the consumption of excess free sugar is responsible for many of our health problems. Sugar is found in many forms, including brown sugar, corn sweetener, corn syrup, dextrose, fructose, glucose, high-fructose corn syrup, honey, lactose, malt syrup, maltose, molasses, raw sugar and sucrose (table sugar). The harm from free sugar consumption seems to come predominantly from fructose (fruit sugar), although there is some doubt remaining in the medical literature around how this harm occurs. Here we are talking about free fructose and *not* fructose found in whole fruit and vegetables. Table sugar or 'sucrose', for example, is composed of 50% glucose and 50% fructose. Fructose is a highly toxic compound and if consumed in excess quantities is metabolised, predominantly by the liver, along two different pathways.

One metabolic pathway leads to the production of triglycerides, the main type of fat that is produced when calorie consumption is in excess of energy needs. This excess fat contributes to ill health by increasing body weight and fat deposition in the body organs, including the liver, muscles and pancreas. This leads on to insulin resistance, fatty liver and metabolic syndrome. The other pathway leads to the excess production of uric acid, resulting in an increased risk of kidney stones and gout. Uric acid can also turn off production of nitric oxide, a key substance that helps protect the artery walls from damage and promotes blood flow by dilating the arteries. Fructose and uric acid production can generate free radicals contributing to oxidative stress, a type of cellular stress that damages cells, proteins and even our genes. Fructose can contribute to increased production of advanced glycation end products (AGEs), harmful compounds that are formed when protein or fat combine with sugar in the bloodstream, leading to more oxidative stress and inflammation[79].

Fructose has adverse effects on brain health and metabolism by upsetting the balance of hunger hormones released from the brain and increasing the feeling of hunger. Fructose reduces the production of the hormone leptin from fat cells and makes the body resistant to the effects of this hormone, which is key in telling the brain that a person is full. In the gut, fructose contributes to 'leaky gut' – the loss of integrity of the gut lining – and hence the movement of toxins from the gut into the blood. It also has negative effects on the composition of the gut microbiome. Excess fructose consumption has been implicated in the development of cardiovascular disease, overweight and obesity, type 2 diabetes and certain cancers[79, 80, 81].

Unfortunately, fruit juice when consumed in excess can also cause these negative effects and thus most healthy eating guidelines suggest limiting fruit juice consumption to 150 ml per day. However, fructose when consumed in whole fruit and vegetables is accompanied by fibre and a large array of vitamins, minerals and antioxidants and is not associated with any of these adverse effects.

We now know that the sugar industry actively hid the evidence linking sugar consumption with chronic disease and even went as far as to pay off scientists to conduct studies that found in favour of sugar consumption despite growing evidence to the contrary[83]. Yes, sugar consumption is associated with an increased risk of chronic illness, but that does not mean animal foods are off the hook.

1.12 Plant-based diets are expensive, aren't they?

This is a commonly cited reason given against the widespread adoption of a healthy plant-based diet. However, this is another myth that needs to be dispelled. The trouble is that in many high-income countries, such as the UK and Canada, ultra-processed foods make up around half of the foods consumed[83, 84]. These foods, which are usually high in calories yet nutrient poor, are cheaper than fresh, nutrient-dense produce. In addition, meat, dairy and eggs are heavily subsidised by governments, allowing the food industry to artificially lower prices. In fact, meat and dairy consumption would be financially unviable if it wasn't for subsidies paid for by our tax pounds and dollars.

Studies have examined the cost of improving the quality of diets. For example, one study examined the cost of the current UK diet against the expected cost if citizens actually followed the national dietary guidelines: the Eatwell guide. These guidelines recommend that around three quarters of the diet should be plant-based and is very supportive of vegetarian and vegan diets. The results found that meeting the recommendations of the Eatwell guide would cost £5.99 per adult per day, which was very similar to the cost of the current diet at £6.02[86].

A study from the US which examined the association of diet quality and spending on food in 78,191 participants in the Nurses' Health Study found that those with the best quality diet spent 24%

more than those with the lowest quality diet[87]. Nonetheless, when the cost of a healthy meat-based diet was compared with the cost of a healthy plant-based diet with extra-virgin olive oil, using the cost of food in the US, the plant-based diet came out top, costing less whilst providing more portions of fruit, vegetables and whole grains[88].

We do have to be mindful that those of lower socio-economic means have to use a greater proportion of their salary than those on higher incomes in order to achieve an equivalent high-quality diet. For example, in a 2020 report on the state of the food system in the UK, it was found that the poorest 20% of households would need to spend 39% of their disposable income on food to meet the cost of the Eatwell guide. This was compared with only 8% of income for the richest 20%. The report also found that more healthy foods were three times as expensive as less healthy foods per calorie, with the cost of more healthy foods, such as fruit and vegetables, rising over the previous four years whilst the cost of unhealthy foods high in sugar, fat and salt had remained stable at a lower price[89]. Thus, it seems that a healthy diet in general is more expensive than a diet composed of ultra-processed foods, rather than a plant-based diet per se.

One problem that arises is that most people are eating pre-prepared and processed meals and the equivalent plant-based versions are currently more expensive. Prices will only be driven down by increasing demand. For example, in 2020 a beef lasagna from a major supermarket in the UK, Asda, cost 90 pence for one serving and four bacon and cheese British beef quarter-pounders cost £2.50. So, when a person considers becoming plant-based and goes to purchase these familiar meals, they find that Asda is selling a vegetarian lasagna for £2.29 per portion and two vegan burgers for £2.50. In contrast, a plant-based diet composed of minimally processed foods, such as fruit, vegetables, whole grains and beans, can absolutely be affordable when accompanied by a small amount of knowledge and skill. For example, Asda sells 400 grams of canned chickpeas for 33 pence, 400 grams of tinned tomatoes for 28 pence, a kilogram of brown rice for 83 pence and a kilogram of frozen spinach for £1.31. It would therefore be perfectly possible to cook a chickpea curry for two people for under £2.

Canadians face similar issues to those described above. In addition, most fruit and vegetables eaten by Canadians are imported, with a high rate of inflation on food in general. In fact, the food inflation index has been consistently higher over the last 20 years than the general inflation index. Canada's *Food Price Report* (11th edition) forecast on food prices for 2021 suggested a 3-5% increase in the price of foods, including fruit, vegetables, meat and seafood[90].

As always, it is our most vulnerable populations that are affected the most, including those living on low incomes, indigenous peoples and visible minorities. Food insecurity is a complex issue requiring attention from all levels of society. As individuals we can reduce the cost of healthy plant foods by buying in bulk, supermarket own brands, dried beans and pulses, frozen fruit and vegetables in larger quantities, conventional rather than organic, in-season produce and avoiding the newer, more expensive, plant-based convenience foods. When you take into account the significant reduction in the risk of chronic illness when consuming a healthy plant-based diet, this further reduces individual and household costs, such as spending on medicines and doctors' visits, time off work and, of course, the cost to society as a whole[91].

1.13 Do international dietary guidelines support a plant-based diet?

Most major national and international nutrition and dietetic organisations are fully supportive of plant-based diets and recognise that a 100% plant-based diet can meet nutritional requirements for all life stages when adequately planned, whilst helping to maintain optimal health and reducing the risk of chronic disease[50]. Many influential clinical guidelines now also endorse the use of plant-based diets in clinical practice. The 2019 American College of Cardiology guidelines for primary prevention of cardiovascular disease support plant-based diets, including vegetarian and vegan diets, as part of their recommendations[92]. The American Association of Clinical Endocrinologists and American College of Endocrinology recommend a primarily plant-based eating plan as the first line lifestyle intervention for treatment of type 2 diabetes[15]. The American Diabetes Association's consensus on nutrition therapy for diabetes and prediabetes acknowledges that vegetarian and vegan diets are beneficial for the prevention and treatment of diabetes[93]. The World Cancer Research Fund recommends a diet centred around fruit, vegetables, whole grains and beans, whilst minimising or avoiding processed foods, processed meat, red meat and sugary beverages, for cancer prevention and after a diagnosis of cancer[94]. The American College of Lifestyle Medicine's dietary lifestyle position statement for treatment and potential reversal of disease recommends 'an eating plan based predominantly on a variety of minimally processed vegetables, fruits, whole grains, legumes, nuts and seeds'. That is pretty much a whole food plant-based diet.

Country-specific dietary guidelines are also supportive and adaptable to a 100% plant-based diet. The Eatwell Guide in the UK recommends at least two-thirds of the diet comes from plant foods[95]; it recommends beans as a healthy protein source and includes dairy alternatives, including soya drinks. Health Canada's dietary guideline from 2019 is one of the most progressive to date, with three-quarters of the plate derived from whole plant foods and the remaining quarter for protein foods in which plant sources of protein are emphasised over animal sources; in addition, for the first time, dairy has been removed as a food group altogether[96]. The answer to this question is a resounding YES!

Chapter 2

Eating meat

2.1 Isn't animal protein better quality than plant protein?

This is a prevailing myth that is still prevalent in our society today. The main reason for thinking that animal-derived protein *might* be better than plant-based protein is that protein from animal sources is considered 'complete' – that is, it provides enough of each of the nine essential amino acids to meet human requirements, whereas most plant sources of protein have lower proportions of certain essential amino acids. For example, beans tend to be lower in methionine and whole grains and nuts lower in lysine. In addition, animal-derived protein is more easily digested compared with plant proteins, in which the food matrix (the combination of components present in the food) partly impairs digestibility. However, this is now considered an extremely outdated concept. All plant foods contain all essential amino acids and eating a variety of whole plant foods throughout the day or even over a few days, when meeting calorie requirements, will mean that protein requirements are easily met without having to worry about specific food combinations[1]. In fact, the lower quantities of certain amino acids, such as methionine and branched chain amino acids (BCAA), leucine, isoleucine and valine, in plant-derived protein may actually be an advantage as they have been implicated in the development of cancer and type 2 diabetes[2, 3]. The lower content of sulphur-containing amino acids in plant foods, such as methionine and cysteine, results in a lower acid load of the diet and thus less burden on the kidneys[4]. In addition, there are some 'complete' plant sources of protein, including soya, quinoa, chia seeds and buckwheat. Soya in fact provides protein with a biological value similar to that of animal protein[5].

More importantly, several lines of evidence demonstrate that obtaining protein from plant sources rather than animal sources is associated with better health outcomes and can reduce the risk of a number of chronic diseases, including cardiovascular disease, type 2 diabetes and certain cancers, whilst promoting healthy ageing[6, 7, 8, 9]. These studies come from different populations around the world, including the US, Canada, Europe, Japan and China, and the results are very consistent[8, 9, 10, 11]. Overall, more is not better when it comes to protein, but the source of protein is key, with animal-derived protein adversely affecting health. This is particularly true for animal flesh in the form of red and processed meat and poultry, but in some studies even egg protein has been found to contribute to ill health[12]. These studies show that just swapping 3% of total energy in the diet from animal protein with plant-derived protein can have a dramatic impact, significantly reducing mortality from several causes with a risk reduction in the order of 20-40%.

2.2 But doesn't saturated fat cause heart disease? *Time Magazine* said so!

First, let's consider where dietary fat comes from. Saturated fats are solid at room temperature and mainly, although not exclusively, found in animal-derived foods. However, all foods that contain fat have some saturated fat, including plant foods.

For example, nuts and seeds have 1-2 grams of saturated fat per 28 grams and avocado will have around 2 grams of saturated fat per avocado. There are a few plant foods that have significant amounts of saturated fat. These include coconut-derived products, palm oil and cacao butter.

There are four main saturated fats in food:

- Lauric acid found in coconuts;
- Stearic acid found in cheese, meat, poultry, dairy and dark chocolate;
- Palmitic acid found in palm oil, butter, cheese, milk and meat, which is the most common saturated fat;
- Myristic acid found in dairy products, coconut oil and palm kernel oil.

Unsaturated fats as oils are liquid at room temperature. This group is further classified into two categories called monounsaturated fats and polyunsaturated fats. Mono-unsaturated fatty acids (MUFAs) are found predominantly in avocado and olive and canola oils, and polyunsaturated fatty acids (PUFAs) are found in nuts, seeds, seed oils, fish and, to a lesser extent, in meat.

Different fatty acids have distinct biochemical properties and can therefore produce different metabolic and physiological effects with different clinical manifestations. Although, in general, saturated fatty acids are considered less healthy than unsaturated fatty acids, the different saturated fats may have an adverse, beneficial, or neutral effect on health. For example, there is no evidence that stearic acid in chocolate is harmful and, in fact, dark chocolate may have benefits for heart health due to the beneficial flavonoids it contains.[13]

The debate on the impact of saturated fat consumption from meat and dairy on health continues unabated, with those supporting a meat-based diet adamant that saturated fat is not the cause of heart disease and those in the plant-based camp certain that fats from animal sources are the driver of heart disease. As mentioned already, there are many foods in the diet that can increase this risk, but please, have no doubt, diets high in saturated fat *do* increase the risk of cardiovascular disease (CVD)[14]. Saturated fat intake increases LDL-cholesterol levels in a linear fashion. LDL-cholesterol in turn is the single most important factor implicated in the development of heart disease and other CVDs. The pro-saturated fat groups will point out correctly that the public health campaign originating in the US in the 1970s to cut fat from the diet has largely failed to improve the health of the nation or in fact global health. This is partly because we never actually cut down our fat intake and, if we did, we largely replaced fat with sugar and refined carbohydrates, which we now know to be just as detrimental to health as a meat-based diet.

The debate started in the 1960s with the work of Ancel Keys, a physiologist who was on a mission to determine the cause of heart disease. He conducted the Seven Countries Study, which showed a strong correlation between the consumption of saturated fat and heart disease[15]. He did not recommend a low-fat diet as the solution but supported the Mediterranean diet pattern, which is high in unsaturated fats from plant sources and emphasises the consumption of whole plant foods. However, he has subsequently been blamed for the 'low-fat' trend that emerged. In response to the US dietary guidelines recommending the lowering of fat consumption, the food industry globally reformulated many processed foods to be low in fat and instead high in sugar. This substitution was later shown to be just as bad for health as foods high in saturated fat. In fact, at the same time, people were eating more processed foods and meals outside of the home in the form of 'fast foods', which are often high in fat, salt and sugar, and hence the health of many nations has continued to deteriorate.

Two large meta-analyses are often quoted to support the claim that saturated fat is not bad for cardiovascular health[16, 17]. Unfortunately, these studies were flawed. What they actually showed was that reducing saturated fat intake by a very small amount when baseline intake is high, does not benefit cardiovascular health. You need to cut intake by a much larger amount, such as would be achieved on a vegetarian or vegan diet, to demonstrate a benefit. In addition, the studies did not consider what was replacing saturated fat in the diet. If saturated fat is replaced by sugar and refined carbohydrates, rates of heart disease remain high, whereas replacing saturated fat in the diet with unsaturated plant-derived fats and unrefined carbohydrates significantly reduces the risk of heart disease[18].

The debate has been refueled by publication of results from the PURE (Prospective Urban Rural Epidemiology) study. This study is a large, ambitious prospective cohort study of around 140,000 individuals aged 35-70 years from 17-21 countries and five continents, including low-, middle- and high-income countries, residing in more than 600 communities. The study has reported controversial findings, such as diets high in carbohydrates increase the risk of death, whereas higher-fat diets, including saturated fat and dairy consumption, improve health outcomes[19, 20], while at the same time reporting that higher intakes of fruit, vegetables and legumes, foods high in carbohydrates, improve health outcomes[21]. So, how can these conflicting results be explained? Essentially, the results demonstrate that participants from low-income countries have suboptimal calorie intakes, predominantly from refined carbohydrates, lower personal income and less access to healthcare, resulting in worse health outcomes, with the opposite being true for those living in high-income countries, eating more meat and dairy (and hence saturated fat), with higher incomes and better access to healthcare. The impact of socio-economic determinants on health cannot be adequately corrected for. So once again, meat and saturated fat consumption are not vindicated.

More recently, the meat industry has waded in by sponsoring publications suggesting that the data linking meat consumption, particularly red meat, with CVD and of course cancer, have been overstated and the reduction in disease risk with meat avoidance is too small to be of clinical consequence[22, 23]. This could not be further from the truth. On a population and societal level, the impact is huge. A 10% reduction in death from CVD, for example, as reported by one of these papers, would amount to 17,000 fewer deaths per year in the UK and 7,104 fewer deaths in Canada based on 2019 data. These same papers make conclusions such as 'omnivores are attached to meat and are unwilling to change this behaviour when faced with potentially undesirable health effects'[25]. For us, this is not a valid reason to underplay the enormous benefits to health afforded by meat reduction or elimination.

So once again we come back to the facts. Diets high in saturated fat, mainly from meat and dairy, are associated with higher rates of CVD and other chronic diseases. This is in part by causing a dose-related increase in blood cholesterol levels, but also because the saturated fat comes packaged with animal protein (see section 2.1) and is devoid of fibre and phytonutrients. Reducing the consumption of saturated fat from animal foods significantly reduces the risk of CVD. This has been clarified in a 2020 Cochrane review of 15 randomised controlled studies (RCTs) on the topic, which showed that reducing saturated fat intake over the longer term can reduce the risk of experiencing a cardiovascular event by 21%, and the greater the reduction in saturated fat consumption the greater the benefit[26]. Vegans, vegetarians and those following predominantly healthy plant-based diets continue to have significantly lower rates of heart disease, in the order of 25%

reduction, which is in line with the lower blood cholesterol levels achieved[27, 28].

Limiting saturated fat intake is supported by all national and international health and nutrition organisations. This includes the Scientific Advisory Committee on Nutrition in the UK, which reviewed all the best available data and concluded that saturated fat intake *is* directly linked to raised blood cholesterol and an increased risk of CVD, thus the current recommendation to limit intake should not be changed[29]. This is also supported by the current Canada Food Guide which states that 'choosing foods that contain mostly healthy fats instead of foods that contain mostly saturated fat can help lower your risk of heart disease'[30].

2.3 Don't we need red meat to get enough iron?

Iron deficiency is the most common nutrient deficiency in the world and therefore not an issue specific to those consuming a plant-based diet. Iron in plant foods is found in the 'non-haem' form rather than the 'haem' iron form found in meat. People eating a vegetarian or vegan diet generally consume as much iron as, or slightly more than, omnivores. Despite having similar or higher iron intakes, their iron stores are usually lower as haem iron from animal sources is absorbed more efficiently[31]. This may sound problematic but may actually be of advantage when it comes to the prevention of chronic disease though it also may play a role in the small but significant increased risk of anaemia reported in some but not all studies in people avoiding meat consumption[32, 33]. The unregulated absorption of haem iron and its propensity to cause oxidative stress in the body has been associated with an increased risk of various chronic diseases, including CVD[34], cancer[35] and type 2 diabetes[36]. Thus, recommending meat consumption to prevent or treat iron deficiency is not advisable.

Non-haem iron absorption depends upon physiological

need and is regulated in part by iron stores. Its absorption can vary greatly, depending upon both the meal composition and the iron status of the individual. For example, phytates in whole grains and beans, and polyphenols in tea and coffee, can inhibit the absorption of iron from plant foods. However, adding vitamin C, citric acid and other organic acids to a meal will greatly increase iron absorption. By paying attention to combining iron-rich foods (whole grains, legumes, nuts, seeds) with foods rich in vitamin C (fruit, vegetables) you can easily enhance iron absorption from plant foods and meet daily requirements at all life stages[37]. Other ways in which you can reduce the impact of phytates in food are by soaking whole grains and beans before cooking and by fermenting or sprouting these too. Using iron-containing cookware, such as a cast iron pan, is also a useful way to increase iron intake[38]. In addition, avoiding the consumption of tea and coffee an hour either side of a meal is advisable.

2.4 But Maasai people eat high amounts of meat and saturated fat and they are healthy?

The Maasai tribe living in Kenya and Northern Tanzania eat a diet high in meat, milk and blood. It is a high-fat, high-cholesterol diet. Despite this, Maasai people have low rates of chronic disease and have low blood pressure and blood cholesterol levels. So, does this mean that eating meat and dairy is good for us? Researchers set about finding out how a diet high in animal foods could still result in good health. They studied 156 Maasai from Kinyawa, Kenya, to answer this question and analysed their DNA, looking for small differences called single nucleotide polymorphisms (SNPs) that might explain why their unusual diet was not leading to poor health[39]. The results showed that there were indeed genetic differences, which have occurred through selective pressure of their diet, that may explain why despite a diet high in saturated fat and cholesterol, blood cholesterol remains low, as does the risk of heart disease. In addition, the Maasai have persistence of the enzyme lactase, required to digest the main sugar in milk, lactose, thus allowing them to continue consuming milk from other mammals beyond weaning. This is in contrast to most people from sub-Saharan Africa.

It has to be remembered that the Maasai tend to have a short life expectancy of less than 50 years and when autopsy studies have been performed, atherosclerosis in the coronary arteries is indeed present although the occurrence of heart attacks is less evident[40]. This may be down to the fact that they are much more physically active compared to the average person in high-income countries and have a much lower overall calorie intake without the continuous supply of calories. These lifestyle factors may well be of importance to their health outcomes.

2.5 Do red meat and processed meat really cause cancer?

Yes. In 2015 the World Health Organization (WHO) determined that processed meat is a major contributor to colorectal cancer, classifying it as group 1 carcinogen – that is, it causes cancer[41]. Consuming just one hot dog or a few strips of bacon daily increases the risk of colorectal cancer by 18%. The World Cancer Research Fund (WCRF) and the American Institute for Cancer Research (AIRC) have also confirmed this finding[42]. Both the American Medical Association and the American College of Cardiology have recommended that hospitals remove processed meat from menus[43].

At the same time, red meat was classified as a group 2a carcinogen – that is, red meat *probably* causes colorectal cancer[41]. A number of studies have also linked processed and red meat to other cancers, including breast, stomach, pancreatic, prostate and bladder cancers[44, 45, 46]. International cancer guidelines clearly state processed meat and red meat should be limited or avoided to reduce the risk of developing cancer[47]. According to estimates by the Global Burden of Disease Project, an independent academic research organisation, about 34,000 cancer deaths per year worldwide are attributable to diets high in processed meat, and red meat could be responsible for 50,000 cancer deaths per year worldwide[48]. Possible mechanisms include the presence of haem iron (found mostly in red meat), nitrates and nitrites (used to keep processed meat fresher for longer and add colour and flavour), which form N-nitroso compounds in the bowel, and heterocyclic and polycyclic amines (produced when meat is cooked at high temperatures). All of these compounds are thought to be cancer promoting[41].

More recently, both processed and unprocessed red meat consumption has been shown to be associated with a specific type of DNA damage in patients with colorectal cancer, making it more certain that red meat does in fact directly cause cancer[49].

2.6 I understand red meat is not healthy, but chicken is okay, isn't it?

It is true that replacing red meat with chicken or other poultry will have a positive impact on health, albeit small. However, there are better choices to make. The rather outdated advice to eat 'white' rather than 'red' meat to improve cholesterol levels has been shown to be misguided based on the results of a study that tested the effects of different sources of protein on blood cholesterol levels[50]. Participants were randomly assigned to a diet high in protein from red meat, white meat and plants and with high or low amounts of saturated fat. Each participant had four weeks on each diet with a washout period in-between each. The results showed that both red and white meat consumption elevated blood cholesterol levels to a similar degree, independently of saturated fat consumption, whereas the diet composed of plant protein did not elevate blood cholesterol levels. The authors concluded: 'The findings are in keeping with recommendations promoting diets with a high proportion of plant-based food but, based on lipid and lipoprotein effects, do not provide evidence for choosing white over red meat for reducing CVD risk.'

For high blood pressure, a combined analysis from the Nurses' Health Study and the Health Professionals Follow-up Study (HPFS), including more than 180,000 men and women from the US, found that the consumption of any animal flesh significantly increased the risk of developing high blood pressure, including poultry, with the risk increasing with intakes as low as one portion per day[51].

A combined analysis of six prospective studies, including almost 30,000 participants, again from the US, found that higher intakes of processed meat, unprocessed red meat *and* poultry, were significantly associated with a small increased risk of developing CVD, although not an increased risk of dying as such[10]. Yet a prior report using data from the Nurses' Health Study and HPFS showed that swapping as little as 3% animal protein from poultry to plant protein reduced the risk of dying, especially if there was an additional unhealthy lifestyle factor present such as physical inactivity or being overweight[52]. Similarly, a report from the EPIC study (see page 6), including 38,000 participants followed for 10 years, showed that the consumption of all sources of animal protein, including poultry, increased the risk of type 2 diabetes, when compared with vegetable protein consumption[53].

In the EPIC study, poultry consumption has also been linked to the development of lymphoma, a type of cancer of the lymphatic system[54]. It has been hypothesised that a cancer-causing poultry virus may be implicated in the association, but this has not been proven. Poultry consumption in some studies has been linked to weight gain and this effect may be even greater than the association with processed and red meat consumption[55].

As you can see, chicken is not given a green card here. Yes, it *may* be better than eating red and/or processed meat, but removing chicken from the diet and replacing it with whole plant foods and healthy sources of protein, such as beans and nuts, is going to significantly reduce the risk of common chronic diseases and lower the risk of dying.

2.7 How does meat cause ill health?

We know of so many reasons why and how eating meat increases the risk of chronic illness. The impact of meat consumption can be divided into the following main categories:

- inflammation
- oxidative stress
- unhealthy gut microbiome
- dyslipidaemia (high cholesterol and triglycerides)
- elevated levels of growth hormones (IGF-1 and oestrogen).

A review of these mechanisms would be a book chapter in itself, so we will summarise here for brevity.

Oxidative stress

Oxidative stress is an imbalance between the normal cellular processes of oxidation and reduction and is a result of the generation of metabolic products known as 'reactive oxygen species' (ROS). Certain 'stressors' can lead to increased levels of ROS, including cigarette smoking, medication, pesticides, radiation and also our diet choices. Oxidative stress then leads to the damage of proteins, DNA and cell membranes. The body requires antioxidants to counter the effects of these damaging ROS. Plant foods contain hundreds of antioxidant compounds and have vastly higher antioxidant content than animal-derived foods[56]. These antioxidants come in two broad categories: carotenoids and bioflavonoids. Both are large groups of structurally related compounds that help plants cope with radiation exposure from sunlight. Studies consistently show that those eating a predominantly plant-based diet have higher levels of antioxidants in the body compared with omnivores[57]. In contrast, compounds within animal-derived foods, such as haem iron (found in haemoglobin and myoglobin in meat) and nitrates and nitrites (found in processed meat) are pro-oxidants, creating oxidative stress and contributing to cellular damage.

Advanced glycation end products (AGEs)

AGEs are a group of compounds that induce oxidative stress. They are formed by a spontaneous chemical reaction between sugars and protein, fats or nucleic acids. Some AGEs are produced in the body every day. However, diet is the biggest contributor to AGE formation (along with tobacco products). AGEs from food are generated more readily from protein-rich foods, when cooking at high temperatures, for longer and with dry heat cooking. Foods that generate the most AGEs are fried and processed foods and also animal-derived foods – meat, dairy, fried eggs. Plant foods such as fruit, vegetables, whole grains and legumes, generate the least amounts of AGEs.

These compounds accumulate over time and have been shown to increase the risk of a number of chronic diseases, including type 2 diabetes, kidney failure, dementia, cancer and atherosclerosis[58, 59].

Unhealthy gut microbiome

This term refers to the adverse changes within the gut microbiome (the trillions of organisms that live in the gut). We understand most about the bacteria within our gut, but there are also viruses, fungi and protozoa present. Dietary choices impact the health of the gut bacteria, which rely predominantly on fibre derived from whole plant foods. Plant-based diets increase bacterial diversity and promote the generation of short chain fatty acids (SCFAs), such as butyrate, propionate and acetate. These SCFAs are signaling molecules that are required for the integrity of the gut lining, maintaining the gut's immune system, reducing colonic pH and protecting against pathogens.

Diets that are deficient in plant-derived fibre, which is the case for most Western-style meat-based diets, are known to result in reduced production of SCFAs and increased production of secondary bile acids (formed by the action of gut bacteria on primary bile acids, which are produced by the liver). Secondary bile acids can damage the gut cells, increase gut permeability and are implicated in the development of cancers of the gastrointestinal tract[60].

Diets high in saturated fat also increase the permeability of the gut lining and allow inflammatory substances, such as bacteria and lipopolysaccharides (bacterial endotoxins), into the circulation, which then contribute to inflammation[61].

An unhealthy gut microbiome has been implicated in virtually every single chronic illness from heart disease to inflammatory bowel disease to type 2 diabetes. One example of how this can occur is through the generation of TMAO (trimethylamine oxide) from gut bacteria that convert choline and carnitine in eggs and meat to TMA (trimethylamine), which later is converted by the liver to TMAO. TMAO generation is associated with the development of atherosclerosis, hence heart disease and stroke, type 2 diabetes and kidney failure[62, 63, 64, 65]. TMAO levels are significantly lower in those consuming more plant foods[64]. It is unclear at present, however, if TMAO is in fact causative in the development of chronic diseases and increased mortality, or represents a confounding factor reflecting a poor quality diet[66]. Nonetheless, it seems beneficial to keep levels as low as possible.

Lipotoxicity/dyslipidaemia

An unhealthy diet, high in saturated fat and processed foods, results in accumulation of fat. This fat is mainly noticed in subcutaneous tissues as people put on weight, but it is the fat that is deposited in the organs – visceral fat – that is most harmful to health. Fat can accumulate in the cells of the muscle, liver, heart and pancreas, causing these organs to become dysfunctional and resulting in metabolic diseases[67]. Fat accumulation in muscle and liver cells leads to insulin resistance and type 2 diabetes.

Fat accumulation can also damage cells and tissue, resulting in cell death, for example in the pancreas, which then can't produce enough insulin. Fat within cells causes mitochondrial dysfunction. Mitochondria are the powerhouses of the cells and dysfunction of these organelles has been associated with a number of chronic diseases.

Accumulation of fat and being overweight puts the body in a continuous state of chronic inflammation as the fat tissue generates inflammatory proteins and growth factors, such as oestrogen and insulin-like growth factor 1 (IGF-1). This in turn contributes to chronic disease, including cancers, which are stimulated to grow by the release of these growth hormones[68]. It is worth noting that you do not have to be overweight or have excess subcutaneous fat to have excess visceral fat. This is why people of normal weight can also develop type 2 diabetes if exposed to a Western-style diet pattern.

Altered hormone levels

Our diet affects hormone and growth factor levels. IGF-1 is a growth factor that is implicated in the development of a number of cancers. Diets high in animal protein result in increased levels of this growth hormone[69]. Vegans, vegetarians and those following more plant-based diets have lower levels of IGF-1 compared with meat-eaters, which explains in part their lower risk of certain cancers[70]. Similarly, oestrogen levels are higher in those consuming the most meat and may be a reason why meat (and dairy) consumption is associated with a higher risk of hormone-related cancers, such as breast and endometrial[44, 71, 72].

2.8 Don't athletes require meat protein for muscle growth?

We have already discussed how animal protein (and fat) can have detrimental effects on health and this is no different for athletes. Yes, protein intake is important for muscle growth, maintenance and repair but again it comes down to choosing the best quality protein. Plant protein wins hands down over animal protein in this regard. In part, this is because plant protein comes packaged with nutrients that are beneficial for preventing injury and enhancing recovery from exercise, such as antioxidant and anti-inflammatory compounds, which are mostly absent from animal sources of protein[56]. In fact, animal protein causes inflammation in the body, which is certainly not an ideal situation for optimal athletic performance[73]. In addition, plant-based sources of protein are also high in healthy carbohydrates, including fibre, and healthy fats, which all help to keep our vital organs functioning to their best ability, clearly crucial for optimal performance. Beans, nuts and seeds can provide all the protein necessary for all types of athletic performance without reaching for protein powders.

Studies have examined whether plant sources of protein can help build muscle as effectively as animal protein. A meta-analysis showed soya protein was as effective as various sources of animal protein for building muscle mass and strength in response to resistance training, but of course without increasing the risk of heart disease and cancer[74].

Small studies of short duration have also been conducted specifically in vegans. One study directly examined the heart function by echocardiography and maximum oxygen consumption of vegan and omnivore amateur runners, with 22 participants in each group, and reported better heart function and cardiorespiratory fitness and endurance, suggesting an advantage for the vegan group[75].

Another study in young, physically active women tested endurance and muscle strength in 28 vegans and 28 omnivores and reported better exercise performance in the vegan group with no disadvantage for muscle strength[76]. A further small study investigated the impact of protein source on muscle mass and strength[77]: 19 vegan and 19 omnivorous men undertook 12 weeks of supervised resistance training. Their protein intake was adjusted to obtain 1.6 grams per kilogram per day, including from protein supplements, either soya or whey. Various measures of muscle mass and strength, including muscle biopsies, were performed at the beginning and end of the study. The results showed that both groups had equal gains in muscle mass and strength, demonstrating that plant protein is not inferior to animal sources of protein.

The suggestion is that the higher carbohydrate intake in a vegan diet and resulting higher glycogen stores may be the reason for the better endurance and performance. Plant-based diets improve endothelial function and hence vascular function, helping to better oxygenate tissues and muscle. The lower blood viscosity due to the better blood lipid profile also enhances blood flow to the muscles[78].

For all athletes who want to achieve optimal performance, planning, knowledge and skills when it comes to nutrition are important regardless of the chosen diet pattern. The increasing number of elite athletes who have adopted a plant-based diet and demonstrated incredible athletic performance is proof in itself. To name just a few: Kate Strong (who has written our

Foreword), Fiona Oakes, Robert Cheeke, Lewis Hamilton, Morgan Mitchell, Kendrick Ferris and Derrick Morgan. Seba Johnson and Nimai Delgado have never eaten meat.

2.9 Doesn't eating meat make men more manly?

Another dominant narrative is that men *need* to eat meat to be manly. The meat industry promotes their products by showing men with large muscles and lots of hair, appearing masculine and seductive whilst eating meat. Needless to say, the science does not support this narrative. Testosterone levels in those eating plant-based diets have been studied and no difference in levels has been found between those eating and not eating meat[79, 80]. None at all.

Testosterone is the main hormone that results in male characteristics. The main factors affecting levels are being overweight and getting older, which both lower testosterone levels. A diet high in fried and processed foods can result in lower levels of testosterone[81]. In fact, the exposure to oestrogen from the consumption of milk from pregnant cows can reduce testosterone levels in men[82]. A healthy plant-based diet can increase manliness because men on this diet are less likely to suffer erectile dysfunction, often one of the first signs of heart disease[83, 84].

Heart disease and cancer are the main killers of men around the world. The arteries in the pelvis and penis are affected by atherosclerosis in the same way as the arteries surrounding the heart. Due to their small size, symptoms of erectile dysfunction occur earlier than those of heart disease. Medication used to treat heart disease can also have the side-effect of erectile dysfunction. In addition, plant-based diets may reduce the risk of prostate cancer in men, with studies showing that removing dairy and replacing it with soya milk is especially important[85, 86, 87].

Treatments for prostate cancer, such as surgery, radiotherapy and anti-androgen medication, can often result in impotence. So, ditch the meat (and dairy) and load up on plants.

2.10 But grass-fed organic meat is healthy, isn't it?

Although there is general consensus that plant-based diets are optimal for health there continues to be a misguided narrative that many of the health concerns related to meat consumption are due to those produced within industrialised, intensified farming systems, such as factory farming. This has led many healthcare professionals to advocate for the consumption of organically reared animals, fed on forage-based diets.

There are indeed some differences in the nutrient profile of organic and non-organic meat, mainly in respect to fatty acid content, with higher levels of the more healthful poly-unsaturated omega-3 fatty acids in organic meat[88]. However, there are no convincing data to suggest the consumption of organic meat leads to superior health outcomes when compared with non-organic meat[89]. At the end of the day, the negative health impacts are due to the animal protein and saturated fat itself, aspects that are not significantly different in organic meat.

There are some potential advantages with organic meat, including lower use of antibiotics in organic farming, but studies have found that bacterial contamination of organic versus non-organic meat is equivalent, although organic meat may have less contamination with antibiotic-resistant bacteria[90, 91]. There are some studies that show those consuming organic foods in general may be healthier, but these results are confounded by factors such as those eating organic food are also consuming more plant foods, less processed meat, less sugar-sweetened beverages and alcohol, and are likely to be of a higher socio-economic status with healthier lifestyles[92].

Eating organic plant foods certainly results in lower exposure to pesticides and herbicides, but whether this translates into better health outcomes in humans is not yet certain[93]. Two studies to date have suggested a lower risk of certain cancers in those consuming the most organic foods (animal and plant-based foods), which may be related to lower pesticide exposure[94, 95]. However, the vast majority of our exposure to environmental toxins comes in the form of persistent organic pollutants (POPs). These toxins come from consumption of animal-derived foods, including fish and dairy, as POPs concentrate higher up the food chain, mainly in fat[96]. POPs pose a risk to human health due to the increased risk of type 2 diabetes[97], certain cancers[98] and CVD[99]. Studies have shown that organic meat has equivalent amounts of POPs when compared with non-organic meat[100], with some studies showing that levels of environmental contaminants are in fact higher in organic meat[101]. What seems more certain is that choice of dietary pattern is of greater importance when it comes to exposure to POPs, with higher blood levels in those consuming the most meat and high-fat animal foods, with vegetarians having lower levels of POPs compared with meat eaters[102, 103, 104].

2.11 What about all the new plant-based meat alternatives – are they healthy?

We believe that plant-based meat alternatives (PBMA) are better for the environment than eating animal meat and certainly better for the animals. However, to date there is very little data on the human health impacts[105]. It has been suggested that these PBMAs are 'healthier' as many are lower in saturated fat, devoid of cholesterol and inflammatory animal protein and some even contain fibre. However, most are still considered ultra-processed foods, often high in sodium and some processed ingredients and hence pale in comparison with whole plant foods such as beans and lentils.

A diet high in processed and refined plant-based foods has been shown to be as detrimental to health, if not more so, than an animal-based diet[27, 106]. In addition, some of the newer products contain ingredients that have not previously been used in food, such as haem iron from soya nodules, so their impact on health is of course unknown. Having said that, there is a great variation in the available PBMAs, with some that have been used in traditional vegetarian diets, such as tofu, tempeh and seitan, being healthy additions to the diet and a very different proposition from the newer ones that attempt to imitate the taste and texture of actual meat[107].

Scientists are on the case and have begun to investigate the health impact. At the time of writing there has only been one well designed study comparing PBMAs with meat, which measured body weight and a number of markers in the blood that relate to the risk of CVD[108]. The main aim of the study was to examine the differences in blood levels of TMAO (trimethylamine oxide) after eight weeks of eating PBMAs compared with animal meat. The other outcomes measured were differences in blood IGF-1 concentrations, metabolic markers (blood lipids, glucose and insulin), blood pressure, weight and microbiota composition.

The study randomly assigned 36 participants to consume two or more servings per day of PBMAs or meat for eight weeks each and then crossed over to do the opposite, while keeping all other foods and beverages as similar as possible between the two phases. All PBMAs were supplied by Beyond Meat. All meat products were supplied by a San Francisco–based organic foods delivery service; the red meat sources were grass-fed, organic.

The results showed that, compared with the animal meat, PBMAs led to significant reductions in levels of TMAO and

LDL-cholesterol and a reduction in body weight. Fasting concentrations of IGF-1, insulin, glucose, HDL-cholesterol, and triglycerides, and blood pressure, were not significantly different between the two phases of the study.

Of course, one can always be sceptical about these results given that the study was funded by an unrestricted grant from Beyond Meat. In its defence, the study was well designed and Beyond Meat was not involved in the study design or analysis of the data. The study compared PBMAs with animal-based meat, so they chose to compare like with like as much as possible. They could have biased the results by comparing PBMAs with processed meats like bacon, sausage and deli meats for example, but instead chose to compare them with organic, grass-fed meat which would, at least in theory, give 'better results' than factory farmed or processed meat. The results are also entirely plausible based on what we know about the impact of diet on health. So, all in all, these are encouraging results.

There have been several clinical studies conducted on the meat substitute Quorn, available in many countries around the World (although not North America) and first approved in the UK. Quorn is made from mycoprotein, which is produced when an aerobic microfungus converts carbohydrate into protein. Quorn is high in fibre and protein and low in fat, including saturated fat. The type of fibre is of interest as two-thirds of it is beta-glucan, which has been associated with several specific health benefits. Studies suggest that Quorn may have benefits for promoting satiety, lowering cholesterol, glucose and insulin regulation and can stimulate muscle synthesis[109].

As with all aspects of diet, some PBMAs will be better than others but common sense tells us that the best diet is one composed of minimally processed whole plant foods and these newer processed PBMAs should be kept to a minimum in the diet and used as 'an occasional food' or transition food only. We also need to be mindful of the fact that the main driving force behind PBMAs (and also cultured 'meat') is the corporate food system and their industry profits and not concerns for human health. The huge investment in these new products from so-called 'philanthropists' is diverting money away from small-holder crop farmers globally who are struggling to make a living and will ultimately mean that our food system is not in the hands of farmers but remains at the mercy of 'Big Food'.

Chapter 3

Eating dairy

3.1 Don't we need dairy for calcium to maintain bone health?

In Western countries, dairy products provide a significant source of dietary calcium, and hence there remains ongoing concern about sufficiency of calcium from a diet that excludes dairy. Nonetheless, calcium is a mineral found in soil, which is absorbed into the roots of plants, so it is present not only in the grass that cattle eat, but in many plants we humans eat. No other animal on this planet consumes milk after weaning and certainly not from another species.

Calcium is a nutrient required for bone health, but there is no scientific evidence that consuming dairy improves bone health or prevents osteoporosis. The truth is quite the opposite. Countries that consume the most dairy milk actually have the highest rates of bone fractures[1]. What is more important for bone health together with calcium intake is regular weight-bearing exercise, adequate vitamin D and the abundance of nutrients obtained from eating plenty of fruit and vegetables[2].

Cows obtain calcium from plant sources, including grass. Thus, for humans, a diet which incorporates low-oxalate green leafy vegetables, legumes, calcium-set tofu (where extra calcium is added in the manufacturing process), nuts and seeds provides sufficient quantities of calcium. Once concern raised is regarding oxalate in plant foods, which is an organic acid found in plants that can bind calcium in the gut and reduce its absorption. Examples of high-oxalate greens include spinach and chard. Of note though, the bioavailability (the amount absorbed) of calcium from low-oxalate green vegetables, such as bok choy, broccoli and kale, is higher than that from dairy. In addition, plant-milks are often fortified with calcium in similar quantities to that found in cow's milk.

Country-based guidelines vary in the recommended daily amount, from 700 milligrams per day for adults in the UK to 1000 in North America. There is increasing recognition amongst the healthcare community that dairy consumption is not essential for human health as there is very little evidence that it improves any health-related outcome[3]. In fact, lactose malabsorption is very common, affecting 50–95% of people in many non-Caucasian populations, and can lead to distressing abdominal symptoms[4]. Lactose, the main sugar in milk, is a disaccharide composed of galactose and glucose sub-units. We need the enzyme lactase, in the small intestine, to break it down into these sub-units to be absorbed into the bloodstream. If it persists in the intestine undigested, lactose will ferment, leading to the symptoms of lactose intolerance. Interestingly lactose intolerance can develop at any age.

Bone health is, of course, an important consideration with any diet pattern, including one that is plant-based. A healthy diet and lifestyle are fundamental to preventing osteoporosis later in life. Important nutrients for bone health, in addition to calcium, include protein, potassium, magnesium, folate and vitamin K, which can all be obtained from a healthy vegan or vegetarian diet, and vitamin D (from sunlight or supplement)[5].

Some concerns have rightly been raised about bone health in those following a vegetarian and vegan diet. A systematic review and meta-analysis of 20 studies including 37,134 participants examining bone mineral density and fracture risk, found that vegetarians and vegans had lower bone mineral density and vegans an increased risk of fracture compared with omnivores[6]. The main limitation of the study, and hence its applicability, is that in only one of the 20 studies was diet quality taken into consideration. In that one study there was no adverse effect of a vegetarian or vegan diet on bone mineral density. Diet quality is important as simply being vegetarian or vegan does not automatically imply a healthy eating pattern. Rather it tells us what is not eaten in terms of animal products but not what is being eaten, which could be a nutrient-dense diet rich in whole plant foods or one that is heavy in processed food.

More recently, an updated analysis from the EPIC-Oxford study (section 1.4) reported an increased risk of bone fractures in those consuming a vegan diet[7]. Of note, the first report from the same study cohort published in 2007 showed no differences in the self-reported incidence of fractures between meat eaters, fish eaters and lacto-ovo-vegetarians, but vegans had a 30% higher risk of fracture compared with meat eaters[8]. However, when the results were adjusted for calcium intake, those consuming at least 525 milligrams of calcium per day, regardless of diet pattern, showed no increase in risk of fracture, suggesting that if the diet contains an adequate amount of calcium there is no disadvantage for bone health on a plant-based diet.

The more recent analysis has shown an increased rate of fracture in those not consuming meat. This was not exclusive to vegans and included vegetarians and fish eaters, but the effect was more pronounced in the vegan group. For vegans the impact was greatest for hip fractures, with a 231% elevated risk compared with meat eaters. Vegans had a 43% increased risk of developing any fracture compared with meat eaters. In absolute terms, this amounted to 19 more cases of fractures in vegans for every 1000 people over 10 years.

The points of interest are that body mass index (BMI) had a major influence on fracture risk, with a BMI of less than 22.5

associated with the increased risk. For vegans with a BMI greater or equal to 22.5, this risk disappeared. This association between BMI and fracture risk is well-known, as carrying more weight increases bone density and also provides better 'cushioning' if you have a fall[9]. The fracture risk was also only increased in women (who made up more than two-thirds of the participants) and not men. Vegans in this study had a lower than recommended intake of calcium and a lower use of hormone replacement therapy in women compared with meat-eaters, factors that are relevant to the risk of bone fractures. The mean calcium intake for vegans was around 600 milligrams per day, so not meeting UK recommendations for 700 milligrams per day.

We also know from prior reports from the EPIC-Oxford cohort that the vegans had lower B12 and vitamin D intakes compared with the non-vegans[10]. Only around 50% of vegan participants in this study were taking dietary supplements, which meant that 50% were relying on food sources of vitamin B12 and vitamin D, which we know are inadequate. These participants were recruited in the 1990s at a time when fortification of plant-based alternatives was not common and knowledge and information on healthy vegan diets was less accessible. Major limitations are that the study cannot tell us the cause of the fractures, if they were due to poor bone health or to accidents, and the study did not correlate fracture rates with vitamin D status, a major factor in bone health.

A subsequent report from the Adventist Health Study 2, which included more than 96,000 Adventists from North America who had been followed since 2002, reported that vegans had a 55% increased risk of developing a hip fracture compared with omnivores[11]. Again, this figure sounds alarming but, in absolute terms, amounts to 1.5 extra hip fractures per 1000 vegans per year. Again, the increased risk was only seen in women, not men, and this time the risk completely disappeared in vegans taking both calcium and vitamin D supplements with intakes of calcium of around 1000 milligrams per day.

These studies highlight that a plant-based diet should be well-planned to ensure it is providing all the nutrients we know support bone health. In addition, we should prioritise weight-bearing and muscle-strengthening exercises and avoid foods and lifestyle habits that adversely affect bone health. This includes excess salt consumption (usually from processed and packaged foods), caffeine, alcohol, sugar-sweetened beverages especially those with phosphoric acid, and smoking. Maintaining a BMI in the middle of the normal range may also be advisable, rather than being 'too thin'.

We must not forget that both the EPIC-Oxford and Adventist Health studies have shown us that a vegan diet is associated with at least a 50% reduction in risk of high blood pressure, significantly lower levels of blood cholesterol, a 25–30% reduction in ischaemic heart disease (this includes vegetarians as well), 15% reduction in cancer risk and at least a 50% reduction in risk of type 2 diabetes in those not eating meat[12]. These are all major causes of death and disability and a far greater risk to personal and public health than bone fractures.

Returning to the topic of dairy and bone health it's worth noting that the 2019 official dietary guidelines for Canada removed dairy as a food group given its non-essential nature, its exclusion of communities of colour who are more likely to have lactose malabsorption, and the harmful impact of dairy farming on the environment[13]. Let's hope other countries' guidelines follow suit.

3.2 Don't we need dairy for iodine?

Iodine deficiency remains a major global public health concern, affecting around two billion people worldwide[14]. This is not a unique problem for those consuming a plant-based diet. Iodine is naturally found in sea and soil. However, unless close to the sea, the iodine content of soil is generally low and hence most plant foods are not a good source.

Iodine is required to produce thyroid hormones. Thyroid hormones are required for brain development and iodine deficiency is the most common preventable cause of brain damage[15].

Omnivores obtain iodine indirectly from dairy and, of course, from fish. Dairy contains iodine because cows' feed is supplemented with iodine and also because of the contamination of milk with iodine from the iodophors used in milking machine sanitation[16]. Fish absorb iodine from seawater and their diet. There is also some iodine in eggs, predominantly because it's added to chicken feed. There is no easy way of knowing how much iodine is present in whole plant foods. Seaweed is a source of iodine and salt is iodised in many countries such as North America to reduce the risk of deficiency. So, for all diet patterns the key is to know where you are obtaining iodine from. For those on a plant-based diet options include plant milks, which are increasingly being fortified with iodine, iodised salt (less desirable given the negative impact of excessive salt consumption), seaweed or a supplement. A supplement is likely the best option during pregnancy and lactation when adequate iodine intake is crucial.

3.3 I have heard that dairy can cause cancer. Is this true?

There are sound theoretical and mechanistic reasons why dairy consumption might increase the risk of cancer. The aim of a mammal's milk is to promote the growth of their young and therefore cow's milk and other dairy products are high in growth hormones such as IGF-1. Diet and lifestyle factors have a significant impact on the level of IGF-1 in the blood, with higher levels associated with an increased risk of cancer[17]. Cows are usually artificially inseminated to be pregnant at the same time as lactating to increase their productivity and hence dairy is high in female hormones such as oestrogen and progesterone. These hormones are implicated in increasing the risk of female cancers, such as breast, ovarian and endometrial cancers[18, 19]. In the laboratory, casein, the main protein in milk, has been shown to increase the growth of cancer cells[20].

Another concerning finding is the presence of bovine leukaemia virus in breast cancer cells, with the suggestion that this virus, acquired from consuming 'food' from infected cows, may increase the risk of developing breast cancer[21, 22].

The scientific data on dairy and risk of cancer in humans is mixed and it is difficult to be conclusive. This is because we don't eat foods in isolation and the quality of the overall diet pattern is more important than the individual components. If someone is consuming dairy instead of fruit and vegetables, then their health will suffer. But if dairy is eaten instead of red and processed meat, then it may appear that dairy is beneficial. Studies have shown that dairy consumption can both increase and decrease the risk of certain cancers. This is why the World Cancer Research Fund (WCRF) does not make specific recommendations on the consumption of dairy in their guidelines on cancer prevention. For example, dairy consumption has been linked to a lower risk of colorectal cancer (bowel cancer)[23]. This is predominantly because of the calcium content of dairy which acts to neutralise the negative impact of secondary bile acids in the gut, compounds that are more readily formed when eating the standard Western-style diet. Of course, calcium from dairy can be replaced by plant sources of calcium, and the impact of doubling fibre intake from the average 18 grams per day to nearer 40 grams is far greater than that of calcium, having the potential to halve the incidence of colorectal cancer[24].

The strongest evidence for the link between dairy and cancer comes from studies in prostate cancer[25]. In a combined analysis of 32 different studies, 400 grams of dairy intake per day (equivalent to around 400 millilitres of milk) increased the risk of prostate cancer by 7%. Some of this risk may be from higher intakes of calcium, which is thought to increase the risk of prostate cancer through reducing circulating vitamin D levels[26]. In addition, evidence points to higher exposure to IGF-1 through dairy consumption, with independent studies showing that higher levels of IGF-1 in the blood increases the risk of prostate cancer by 38%[27]. IGF-1 levels in vegans are lower compared with non-vegans[28].

Focusing in on prostate cancer, we know from a seminal randomised study by Dr Dean Ornish, that a low-fat plant-based diet along with other healthy lifestyle habits can arrest, and in some cases reverse, the progression of early stages of prostate cancer[29]. Dr Ornish went on to show the mechanisms by which his intervention might have been working, by lengthening the telomeres (caps at the end of the chromosomes) and significantly changing gene expression in prostate biopsies collected before and after the intervention[30, 31]. A further study has confirmed that a healthy plant-based diet, as defined by the plant-based diet index (see section 1.4 for more on this index) is associated with significantly lower PSA levels, a marker of prostate health in men, which becomes elevated in cases of prostate cancer[32].

There is some suggestive evidence that dairy consumption may increase the risk of 'female'-specific cancers, with the strongest evidence for endometrial cancer and mixed data on breast cancer[3]. Nevertheless, there are better choices to make. Replacing cow's dairy with soya milk and foods can reduce the risk of breast cancer[33]. For example, regular consumption of tofu can reduce the risk of breast cancer by around 22% when comparing those who eat the most versus those who eat the least[34]. One study found that swapping soya milk for dairy milk could reduce the risk by up to 32%[35]. The other interesting feature of this study was the finding of a dose response – that is, the higher the daily consumption of dairy milk, the higher the associated increased risk of breast cancer. A finding of a dose response in studies lends more weight to causation rather than association, like that found in similar types of study looking at smoking and lung cancer. Consuming soya in childhood and adolescence can even reduce the risk of developing breast cancer later in life[36]. Similar findings are true for prostate cancer where soya milk and foods are associated with a lower risk[37]. Fortified soya and pea milks have a similar amount of protein and calcium as cow's milk without the saturated fat and health risks associated with dairy consumption.

3.4 Don't children need milk to develop and grow?

Parents often worry that dairy is required for normal growth and development in childhood. However, when you consider that more than 70% of the world's population have lactose malabsorption after weaning, the inclusion of dairy for most children will result in distressing abdominal symptoms[4]. In fact, dairy consumption is linked to the development of eczema, asthma and acne, conditions that negatively impact a child's quality of life[3, 37, 38, 39]. In addition, cow's milk allergy is the commonest single cause of fatal anaphylaxis in school-aged children in the UK[41]. Even though children who include dairy in their diet may grow to be taller, by approximately 1.5 cm, this may actually be a disadvantage as greater height has been shown to increase the risk of developing cancer[41, 42]. (Some studies also show an increased risk for heart disease with height but data are more mixed.)

Did you know that cow's milk consumption in infants and toddlers increases the risk of iron deficiency in children? This is because cow's milk has a low iron content, increases blood loss from the gastrointestinal tract and calcium and casein inhibit the absorption of iron from plant foods[44]. It is therefore a common recommendation to avoid dairy consumption in children who are iron deficient or at risk of developing this.

Another devastating effect of cow's milk consumption is an increased risk of type 1 diabetes, a condition whose incidence is rising and starts in childhood. It is thought that in genetically susceptible individuals, exposure to cow's milk protein is a key environmental trigger. This is because the body mounts an immune reaction to cow's milk protein, forming antibodies to this foreign protein. These same antibodies can cross-react with cells in the pancreas, which get caught up in the crossfire, leading to the loss of insulin-producing pancreatic β-cells and the development of type 1 diabetes. The earlier that cow's milk is introduced into the diet the higher the risk of developing type 1 diabetes[45]. The science is by no means clear cut on this topic but for us the precautionary principle must apply[46]. Given that there is absolutely no requirement for cow's dairy in the diet, avoiding exposure is the sensible approach. For mothers who require an infant formula, the use of soya formula has a long history of safety and is the best alternative when breastfeeding is not possible[47].

3.5 Yoghurt and cheese can help the gut microbiome, so won't I miss out on these benefits?

Most cheeses (although not all) and dairy yoghurts are fermented milk products that have been made using lactic acid bacteria, such as *Lactobacillus*, *Lactococcus*, and *Leuconostoc*. Fermentation is a food-processing technique that has been used for centuries to increase the shelf-life of food, but it can also increase the digestibility and nutrient content. If the product has been heat-treated or pasteurised after the fermentation process, then the live bacteria are killed off. If this has not taken place then the live cultures consumed have been associated with health benefits by improving the health of the gut microbiome, the 100 trillion micro-organisms, mostly bacteria, living in our gastrointestinal tract. These fermented dairy products with live bacteria are known as 'probiotics'[48].

The enormous wealth of scientific literature on gut health has informed us that the health of the gut microbiota, particularly the bacteria, is crucial to our physical and mental well-being and the microbiome is now considered a vital organ in its own right. A healthy gut microbiome is one that has a diverse range of bacteria in the right proportions, with an abundance of specialised bacteria that produce important molecules called short-chain fatty acids (SCFA). Abnormalities of the gut microbiome have been associated with chronic conditions such as obesity, type 2 diabetes, cancer, inflammatory bowel disease and CVD, to name just a few. Many dietary, lifestyle and environmental factors affect the health of the gut bacteria, with negative effects associated with diets high in saturated fat and sugar and low in fibre, use of antibiotics and other prescribed medications. Positive effects have been shown from eating high-fibre diets and probiotic foods, which contain live bacteria and yeasts. This is where cheese and yoghurt come in to play. The consumption of these foods improves the health of the gut microbiota by increasing healthy bacteria, such as *Lactobacillus* and *Bifidobacteria*, and decreasing less healthy strains such as *Bacteroides* and *Clostridia*[49].

However it is important to emphasise that the fibre content of the diet is the most important determinant of the health of the gut microbiome, along with the diversity of plant foods. Fibre is only found in plant foods and is required for fermentation by the gut bacteria in the colon. This fermentation supports the growth of the specialised bacteria, which is crucial for SCFA production. Without enough fibre, the health of the gut bacteria suffers and, consequently, so does our health. Plant-based diets have been associated with the best gut health and the good news is that it only takes a few days for the healthy gut bacteria to appear when you adopt a plant-based diet[50]. The American Gut Project, a unique crowd-sourced project the goal of which is to better understand the gut microbiome in health and disease, reported that participants who ate more than 30 different types of plant per week had gut microbiomes that were the most diverse and that these bacteria carried fewer antibiotic-resistant genes, a likely consequence of eating less meat[51].

Achieving 30 different plant foods per week is quite hard unless you are eating at least a predominantly plant-based diet. It might be that fermented foods are a useful addition to the diet, but these are easily incorporated in a plant-based diet without having to reach for dairy foods. Examples include tempeh, sauerkraut, kimchi, water kefir, dosa, idli and miso[52, 58].

Chapter 4

Eating eggs

4.1 Eggs are a healthy source of protein, aren't they?

It is common to hear that eggs are a healthy protein source. This stems from the fact that egg whites provide a source of 'complete' protein (discussed in section 2.1) and that this comes packaged with a relatively low saturated fat content when compared with other sources of animal protein. One large egg (50 grams) contains 6 grams of protein and around 1.5 grams of saturated fat when compared with a 70-gram serving of beef which has around 4 grams of saturated fat. Protein can be more satiating than carbohydrate and fat, in part due to differential effects on gut hormones that provide us with signals of fullness, although the science on this topic is mixed and results certainly are not consistent[1, 2]. Nonetheless, when it comes to egg consumption, typically for breakfast, interventional studies (where study participants are allocated to groups which receive different interventions) suggest that eggs are associated with improved satiety compared with breakfasts such as cereal or bagels, which then results in a reduced calorie intake during the remainder of the day[3, 4, 5]. Interestingly, this effect does not seem to be specific to egg protein, or indeed animal sources of protein. When the satiating impact of different protein sources were compared in 12 healthy subjects, it was found that egg albumin, casein, gelatine, soya and pea protein had an equivalent effect[6]. Both Quorn (mycoprotein) and soya have been compared with chicken and shown to be superior in their satiating effects[7]. This suggests that it is not necessarily the egg or animal protein per se that produces satiety, but protein in general. Given the huge benefits to health associated with swapping animal protein for plant sources of protein, it seems tofu scramble is the better breakfast choice[8].

4.2 Eggs are a source of healthy nutrients, aren't they?

Most of the nutrients in eggs are contained in the yolk. These include B vitamins, including vitamin B12, vitamin D, iodine (if added to chicken feed), selenium, biotin, choline, lutein and zeaxanthin (carotenoids)[9]. However, these individual nutrients themselves do not make a food healthy. The whole package and its impact on the body are more important. Eggs come packaged with a sizable portion of cholesterol – around 200 milligrams – and more saturated fat than plant foods, 'nutrients' we don't really want to be consuming.

The more important question to ask is how eggs compare with other foods that contain similar nutrients but different packaging. What would happen to health outcomes if eggs were substituted for another food? Observational studies that have conducted substitution analyses have clearly answered this question. One such large study, including more than 400,000 men and women followed for 16 years, found that just substituting 3% of energy from eggs with plant sources of protein could reduce the risk of dying by 18% to 45% in men and 20% to 39% in women[10]. Another substitution analysis combining the results of six studies and including 29,682 participants followed for around 19 years showed that substituting eggs just once a week with virtually any other foods other than processed meat led to reductions in cardiovascular disease and risk of dying from all causes. When substituting one egg *per day* with whole grains, legumes, nuts or fish, there were even bigger gains, with swapping out eggs for nuts lowering the risk of cardiovascular disease by 21% and the risk of dying from all causes by 22%[8]. These types of substitution study demonstrate that plant sources of protein are better for health than egg whites, often considered to be a healthy source of protein without the harms associated with the consumption of the egg yolk.

One major concern with regard to the body's handling of the nutrients in eggs is related to choline. In people consuming an omnivorous diet, gut bacteria convert choline to trimethylamine (TMA). This is absorbed into the blood and converted into trimethylamine oxide (TMAO), a substance that has been intimately associated with the development of atherosclerosis, heart failure, type 2 diabetes and kidney failure[11, 12, 13, 14, 15]. In contrast, those consuming a 100% plant-based diet do not have the required bacteria to form these substances, and choline from plant foods does not get converted into TMAO[16]. Whether TMAO is actually *causing* these chronic conditions or merely an associated factor reflecting a poor quality diet remains an open question, but it's clear that eating a diet that keeps TMAO levels low may be better for long-term health[13].

The other aspect to consider is food safety, such as the risk of transmission of unwanted substances, whether they are environmental toxins, pollutants or infections. When it comes to eggs, they don't fare well in this regard. In 2018, there were nearly 50,000 cases of foodborne infection in the European Union, with one in three cases caused by *Salmonella*, mainly linked to the consumption of eggs[17]. In Canada, one in eight people (four million Canadians) get sick each year from contaminated food, with over 11,500 hospitalisations and 240 deaths each year due to food-related illnesses, mainly from animal products, of which one in four are due to *Salmonella*[18].

Although eggs may be better for health compared with a bacon sandwich made with white bread, we can make healthier and safer choices by eating plant sources of the same nutrients. For example, an 80 gram serving of tofu has 6 grams of protein and contains choline, selenium and iron whilst being very low in saturated fat and containing no cholesterol.

4.3 What impact do eggs have on blood cholesterol levels?

Another ongoing debate is the impact of dietary cholesterol on health. Given that eggs are high in cholesterol, with a large egg containing around 200 milligrams, they are often used to either defend or refute the claim. Vegans often argue that because eggs are high in cholesterol, they must be a cause of heart disease. It seems that in recent years, dietary guidelines have de-emphasised the harm of dietary cholesterol, with a greater focus on the overall dietary pattern[19]. This does not mean that dietary cholesterol no longer matters; it just means that other components in the diet have a greater impact on health outcomes – namely, saturated fat. The impact of saturated fat consumption in the diet has a far greater and more predictable effect on blood cholesterol levels and hence the risk of cardiovascular disease than does dietary cholesterol[20]. The relationship between saturated fat and blood cholesterol levels is pretty much linear[21]. The more you eat, the higher your blood cholesterol level. This is not the case for dietary cholesterol. If you are already eating a diet relatively high in cholesterol, like the typical Western diet, then adding a bit more won't affect blood cholesterol levels. However, if you are eating a diet free of cholesterol – that is, a vegan diet – then adding an egg or two into your diet *will* raise blood cholesterol levels. The impact of dietary cholesterol from a food like eggs is greater when the diet is already low in cholesterol. At higher intakes of cholesterol, the impact on blood cholesterol plateaus and thus eating more doesn't make a great deal of difference.

Having said all this, it does not mean that dietary cholesterol is healthy or necessary. Our body makes all the cholesterol it needs. You do not need to eat any. Blood cholesterol levels are lowest in those following a vegan or predominantly plant-based diet, especially when the diet is centred around whole plant foods[22]. Omnivores with high blood cholesterol levels can lower levels as effectively as by taking medication by adopting a healthy plant-based diet alone, which is one of the reasons why those eating a plant-based diet have some of lowest rates of heart disease of any diet pattern[23].

So back to the question of eggs. It really depends on the quality of the rest of the diet. Overall, the science shows that up to one egg a day is probably okay but above that level there are detrimental effects on blood lipids. This is on the basis of an updated meta-analysis of 66 randomised studies, so good quality data, demonstrating that egg consumption does indeed elevate blood total and LDL-cholesterol levels[24].

4.4 What impact do eggs have on the risk of cardiovascular disease (CVD) and type 2 diabetes?

A key question is whether egg consumption contributes to an increased risk of chronic illness. The answer is yes, it does. A large analysis combining the results of six studies in which 29,615 adults were followed for a median of 17.5 years showed that each additional half egg consumed per day was associated with a 6% higher risk of CVD and an 8% increased risk of dying from all causes[25]. A further study including 521,120 participants showed that each additional half egg consumed per day increased the risk of dying from CVD, cancer and, indeed, all causes by 7%, and that these negative impacts on health were predominantly due to the cholesterol content of the egg[26].

There is more certain evidence to show that egg consumption increases the risk of developing type 2 diabetes in Caucasian and non-Caucasian populations. In people with type 2 diabetes, eggs cause further harm by significantly increasing the risk of CVD. There have been three meta-analyses assessing the impact of egg consumption on the risk of type 2 diabetes which together confirm an 18-42% increased risk in those eating one or more eggs per day[27, 28, 29]. In addition, in people living with type 2 diabetes, those consuming the most eggs were shown to have a 40% increased risk of CVD[28].

We also need to remember that the interpretation of many studies on eggs is clouded by the fact that they are funded by the egg industry. Despite the studies showing unfavourable impacts on blood lipid levels, those funded by the egg industry appear to considerably downplay these effects, often by using statistical manipulations to produce more favourable results[30].

The bottom line – consumption of eggs is not necessary. The literature can appear confusing and is complicated by industry funding. There is certainly enough data to cause concern regarding the negative health impacts of consuming eggs. We would suggest to you that eggs are best left off the plate.

Chapter 5

Eating fish

5.1 Isn't eating fish good for health?

A 100% plant-based or vegan diet is one of the healthiest diet patterns you can choose and is associated with some of the lowest risks of chronic illness, including cardiovascular disease (CVD), type 2 diabetes, overweight/obesity and certain cancers. So, from the available evidence it can be stated that fish consumption is not necessary in a healthy plant-based diet. But would adding fish to an otherwise healthy plant-based diet improve health further? We don't know the answer to this question as a study comparing a healthy plant-based diet with or without fish has never been done. Most studies that have examined this question within the context of an omnivorous diet have found that eating fish is beneficial to human health[1,2,3]. However, the impact of fish consumption on human health must be considered in the context of the overall dietary pattern and what fish is replacing in the diet. The relevant question is always *'compared to what?'*.

A person eating fish instead of red and/or processed meat will most certainly benefit their health. A person eating fish instead of beans may not. The impact of fish is likely not so much from the fish itself but from what has been removed or replaced from the diet. If you consider this type of substitution analysis, a large study including 85,013 women and 46,329 men from the

Nurses' Health Study (section 1.4) and the Health Professionals Follow-up Study (HPFS, section 1.4) followed for more than 20 years, showed that replacing just 3% of protein from fish with plant protein reduced the risk of dying by 6%[4]. We accept that this is a small effect and has not been replicated in every similar study, but it clearly demonstrates that there are better or equal choices we can make by selecting plant sources of protein.

Fish consumption has been shown to be most beneficial for cardiovascular and brain health. Most of the benefit from fish is attributed to the long chain omega-3 fatty acids, DHA (docosahexaenoic acid) and EPA (eicosapentaenoic acid), present in oily/fatty fish, rather than the whole fish per se. Observational data on fish consumption show that it is associated with a lower risk of heart disease, stroke and death[5]. The proposed mechanism for these findings is that omega-3 fatty acids are associated with a lower heart rate and blood pressure, better endothelial function, lower triglyceride levels and a reduced risk of arrhythmias and hence sudden death.

There have been only two randomised studies of fish consumption in people with heart disease: the Diet and Reinfarction Trial (DART) and the Diet and Angina Randomized Trial (DART-2), both in men[6,7]. The DART study included men who had recently recovered from a heart attack who were asked to consume 200-400 grams of fatty fish a week. The results showed a reduction in death from all causes, which may have been a consequence of the ability of omega-3 fats to reduce the risk of arrhythmias and hence sudden cardiac death. In the DART-2 trial, men with stable angina were randomised to increased fish consumption or fish oil tablets. The results of this study showed a neutral impact of fish consumption but increased risk of death in those consuming the fish oil capsules.

A recent large observational study analysed the impact of fish consumption on CVD risk and mortality in almost 150,000 participants in the PURE study (involving 21 nations,

see section 2.2) who were free from CVD at recruitment[8].
After a median of nine years follow-up, it was found that the
consumption of 175 grams of fish per week (two servings per
week) was *not* associated with a reduction in CVD or mortality.
Interestingly, in the PURE study cohort, fish consumption was
associated with a rise in LDL-cholesterol and fasting glucose,
lowering of triglycerides and no impact on HDL-cholesterol
('good' cholesterol). In contrast, the study went on to analyse
fish consumption in three further cohorts of participants from
40 different nations with known CVD or type 2 diabetes and
showed that 175 grams of fish per week reduced CVD events
by around 13%, CVD mortality by 22%, sudden cardiac death
by 27% and total mortality by 14%. In one cohort the type of fish
was also assessed, and it was the fatty/oily fish (such as salmon,
sardines, tuna and mackerel) that was associated with benefit
whereas other types of fish had a neutral effect. Consuming more
than 175 grams per week did not provide additional benefit. Of
note, there was no analysis provided on cooking methods or the
impact of exposure to environmental pollutants.

Observational studies continue to show a benefit of fish
consumption, around two portions a week, for prevention of
cognitive decline and dementia[9]. However, in the context of a
vegetarian or vegan diet, a report from the Adventist Health
Study examining the impact of animal foods in the diet found
that those consuming meat, including both poultry and fish, had
twice the incidence of dementia compared with those avoiding
meat[9]. Based on a review of all the current data on plant-based
diet and brain health, we accept that more studies are required
before firm conclusions can be drawn[10]. Having said that, many
studies have shown that the beneficial components in the diet
that protect brain health as we age are micronutrients, such as
carotenoids and flavonoids, found in whole plant foods[11, 12]. In
addition, a plant-predominant diet, albeit not 100%, protects
the brain from dementia, in part, by reducing the risk of

cardiovascular risk factors, such as hypertension, type 2 diabetes and high cholesterol, that also increase the risk of dementia[13, 14].

Fish oil and omega-3 fatty acid supplements

Studies of fish oil/long-chain omega-3 fatty acid supplementation have shown variable results, with some showing a benefit and others not. A review in 2019 of 13 randomised studies in participants with CVD risk factors, or already established CVD, showed there might be a benefit of omega-3 supplementation for reducing the risk of heart disease, further heart attacks in those with established disease, and sudden death from arrhythmias (5-12% reduction in risk) but no benefit for the risk of stroke[15]. Having said that, the most recent Cochrane review from 2020 on the topic of long-chain omega-3 supplements and prevention of CVD found that a dose of at least 3 grams per day had little or no effect on all-cause mortality, cardiovascular mortality, cardiovascular events, stroke or arrhythmia[16]. However, the data suggested that increasing long-chain omega-3 intake may slightly reduce coronary heart disease mortality and coronary heart disease events. These effects are very small: 334 people would need to take long-chain omega-3 supplements for several years for one person to avoid dying of coronary heart disease, and 167 people would need to take omega-3 supplements to avoid one person experiencing a coronary heart disease event. The only benefit reported was that long-chain omega-3 supplements might reduce triglyceride levels by 15% in a dose-dependent way. There was also insufficient evidence found to support increasing the consumption of oily fish in the diet for CVD prevention. Similarly, increasing the consumption of short-chain omega-3 fatty acids found in plant foods had a very small benefit only.

Regarding brain health, the 2012 Cochrane review of omega-3 supplements for prevention of cognitive decline and dementia failed to show a benefit[17]. A further review from 2016 also failed to show a benefit for the treatment of mild to moderate Alzheimer dementia[18].

The reason why studies differ in their results is most likely based on variation in the formulation and dose of the supplements and the background rate of fish consumption. In populations that consume fish already, adding omega-3 supplements may not have any further benefit. The opposite may also be true, that omega-3 supplements may benefit those eating little or no fish.

The main caveat to the information presented is that in a select group of people with high levels of triglycerides and who are at high risk of heart disease due to underlying risk factors, or known to have CVD, a large randomised study called the REDUCE-IT study showed that supplementation with a highly purified form of EPA (eicosapentaenoic acid) was able to reduce the chance of death from CVD[19]. However, other studies testing similar hypotheses, but using a combination of DHA (docosahexaenoic acid) and EPA supplementation, have not shown a benefit in patients at high risk of CVD[20, 21]. These discordant results are most likely due to different doses and formulations of omega-3 fatty acids and leave us with uncertainty about the role of supplementation.

A further meta-analysis specifically investigated the impact of EPA supplementation rather than the combination of DHA and EPA, and found a significant benefit for cardiovascular health, suggesting that the type and formulation of omega-3 is key[22]. We would suggest it's always best to have a personalised discussion with your healthcare provider about the benefit of omega-3 supplements based on your medical history and the quality of your diet.

Fish and the Mediterranean diet

The Mediterranean diet, which includes fish, has always been considered a very healthy diet pattern and as of January 2021 has been voted the best diet for four years in a row by a panel of nutrition experts for the *US News and World Report*. So, is it the fish that makes the Mediterranean diet so healthy? It seems not. When researchers studied just this question, the results showed that the most beneficial foods in the Mediterranean diet pattern are the whole plant foods and not fish, which has more of a neutral effect[23]. The Mediterranean diet has been more extensively discussed in section 1.9. For the 10th year in a row, the Ornish diet, which is 100% plant-based, was voted Number One Best Heart Healthy Diet.

5.2 But don't Inuit eat lots of fish and maintain good health?

It turns out this is another nutrition myth and Inuit do get atherosclerosis after all. It has always been believed that their traditional diet, high in marine food and thus omega-3 fatty acids, protected them from atherosclerosis. One study performed CT (computed tomography) scans on two male and two female Inuit mummies – likely to have been between the ages of 16 and 30 years. Cause of death could not be determined but the images clearly demonstrated the presence of calcified atherosclerotic plaques in the carotid arteries, aorta and iliac arteries. Although the cause of atherosclerosis cannot be determined, it is clear that the marine-based diet was not able to protect them from the world's top killer of men and women and atherosclerosis started at a very young age[24]. As is often stated, when choosing a diet, the most important question is: 'Can it keep my heart healthy?' If it cannot, then it is not worth the risk.

5.3 Don't we need to eat fish for omega-3 fats?

Omega-3 fats are important for cardiovascular, brain and eye health[25]. There are three main omega-3 fatty acids. The short-chain omega-3 fatty acid alpha-linolenic acid (ALA) and the two long-chain omega-3 fatty acids – DHA and EPA. ALA is considered essential and must be obtained from the diet; it is found in plant foods. DHA and EPA in most dietary patterns are usually obtained from fish, although fish obtain them from marine algae.

There is an open question as to whether those following a 100% plant-based diet should take a long-chain omega-3 supplement. The body can convert ALA to DHA and EPA but the rate of conversion varies and may reduce with age; it can also differ between individuals based on gender, genetic factors and the overall composition of the diet. Daily requirements of ALA can be met by eating 1-2 tablespoons of chia seeds or ground flaxseeds (linseeds), 2 tablespoons of hemp seeds or 30 grams of walnuts. Some sources do recommend aiming for a higher intake of ALA than the recommended dietary reference intake if consuming a 100% plant-based or vegan diet[26]. It's also important to reduce consumption of omega-6 fatty acids, which if in excess, can interfere with the conversion of ALA to DHA and EPA. These omega-6 fatty acids are mostly consumed in processed oils and processed foods and therefore most people are consuming too much. Aiming for an omega-6 to omega-3 ratio of around 4:1 (as found in flaxseeds, for example) seems optimal[27].

There is evidence to suggest that if DHA and EPA are not being obtained from the diet, there is an increase in the efficiency of conversion from ALA. In the EPIC study (section 1.4), DHA/EPA levels in the blood did not differ as much as expected when comparing fish eaters with non-fish eaters, although levels were lower. However, this confirms that those on a vegan diet do make EPA/DHA. Studies also show that vegans have higher levels of

ALA than omnivores[28]. Having said this, higher levels of EPA/DHA may indeed be beneficial for health based on a combined analysis of 17 studies including 42,466 participants followed for a median of 16 years. Higher blood levels, equivalent to the consumption of around 250 milligrams of EPA/DHA daily, were associated with significant reductions in death from CVD, cancer and all causes[29]. Once again, it is difficult to know how to interpret these results in the context of a 100% plant-based diet, as participants in this analysis were omnivores. We do know from randomised studies that algae sources of omega-3 fatty acids result in a similar rise in blood DHA levels to consuming fish[29, 30].

5.4 Should those on a plant-based diet take an algae-based supplement?

There remains uncertainty as to whether there is a benefit for everyone on a plant-based diet taking DHA/EPA directly so as not to rely on conversion from ALA. This may be particularly important for brain health at the extremes of life. The most reliable source in a plant-based diet would be a micro-algae supplement at a dosage of 250 milligrams DHA/EPA combination per day in adults. Supplementation is certainly recommended during pregnancy and breastfeeding at higher doses if following a plant-based diet as plant-based eaters have been found to have lower circulating levels of DHA/EPA in their blood. It may be prudent for children and older adults also to take a DHA/EPA supplement. Given that we don't yet have a definite answer to this question for all age groups, it is worth keeping up with the science and having an open mind. Until then we will have to make decisions on an individual basis.

5.5 What about the pollutants in fish? Do they affect health?

There are genuine concerns around eating fish because of high levels of contamination by heavy metals such as mercury, environmental and industrial pollutants such as PCBs (polychlorinated biphenyls) and dioxins[31, 32]. The waters that fish now inhabit have become increasingly polluted by the actions of humans on the planet and these pollutants become concentrated, particularly within larger fish. In addition, fish are contaminated with microplastic particles and what is often forgotten is that the fishing industry is itself a major contributor to plastic pollution of our oceans due to the abandonment of fishing gear[33, 34]. Microplastics in the food chain are a source of potentially toxic chemicals such as bisphenol A (BPA), a known endocrine disrupter[36].

We need to apply the precautionary principle here. Just because we have not been able to show conclusive evidence of harm from eating contaminated sources of fish, common sense suggests that avoiding contaminated food should be the default position until safety can be demonstrated. PCBs have been linked to an increased risk of obesity and type 2 diabetes[36, 37]. With rates of cancer on the rise globally, and environmental toxins implicated, it is best in our view to keep exposure to these compounds as low as possible[39]. In addition, there is ongoing concern with regards to mercury exposure to the foetal brain during pregnancy and therefore it is advised that women only consume fish that are relatively low in mercury when pregnant[40].

5.6 But I could eat farmed fish – wouldn't that have less contamination?

Farmed fish, or fish reared by aquaculture, are also not a sustainable or desirable solution (see section 13.6, for the environmental effects). There is a greater problem of pollution created by fish farming, which necessitates the use of chemicals like pesticides, antibiotics, disinfectants and anti-corrosives, to combat the issues of disease and infection, which are easily spread within cramped fish farms[40, 41]. Antibiotics are overused in fish farming, resulting in antibiotic-resistant infections, which ultimately find their way into the human food chain, posing a risk to human health (see section 13.11 for more on antibiotic resistance in animal agriculture). Farmed fish themselves are still contaminated by environmental and industrial pollutants such as PCBs[43]. The nutritional content of farmed fish is also adversely affected by conditions in which they are raised. Farmed fish can have a high fat content, particularly saturated fat and omega-6 fatty acids, and lower levels of omega-3 fatty acids[44].

Conclusion

All in all, it would seem that fish consumption is not *necessary* for heart and brain health. The advantage of a plant-based diet is that it helps prevent heart disease in the first place whereas fish and omega-3 supplements have a very small impact if any on primary prevention. There may be a small advantage of fish consumption or omega-3 supplements for those with established heart disease but it's not clear that this has any advantage over an Ornish-style plant-based diet. Most of the risk factors for dementia overlap with those for heart disease and therefore a plant-based or plant-exclusive diet is expected to be beneficial for brain health too.

Chapter 6

Eating fruit and vegetables

6.1 Isn't too much sugar from fruit bad for you?

This confusion comes from the fact that the main sugar in fruit is fructose. We discussed the problem with consuming too much fructose in section 2.11. However, the fructose in fruit comes packaged with fibre and a mind-boggling array of vitamins, minerals and phytochemicals that are beneficial to health and act to prevent any negative effects of fructose on the body. There is not a single study suggesting that the consumption of whole fruit is bad for health, not even in people with diabetes. The myths that suggest eating too much fruit causes diabetes are just that – myths. There really isn't such a thing as eating too much fruit. When it has been put to the test in small groups of people, even eating 20 portions of fruit a day had no adverse effects and may have had some additional benefits[1].

An analysis of 95 studies examining the impact of fruit and vegetable consumption on risk of dying from cardiovascular disease (CVD) and cancer, our biggest killers, found that there was a significant reduction in risk of death in people consuming at least 10 portions a day[2]. Given that most people in high-income countries are not even meeting the basic recommendation of five portions of fruit and vegetables a day, worrying about eating too much does not seem to be a real concern.

6.2 Why do some health professionals tell people with diabetes to limit fruit consumption?

Nutrition science has been reduced into the study of individual nutrients without considering the whole food. That's why, in some circles, carbohydrates have been vilified as they are all digested to sugar and hence must be the cause of type 2 diabetes! However, carbohydrates are *not* a food group. The healthiest foods on this planet are predominantly composed of carbohydrates: fruit, vegetables, beans and whole grains. Eating unrefined carbohydrates, naturally packaged with fibre and phytonutrients, is associated with some of the lowest rates of chronic disease, and that includes fruit. However, *refined* carbohydrates, including foods that contain white flour and table sugar, are associated with ill health. It is the whole food package that matters, not the individual components. It does not matter if your diet is high-, moderate- or low-carb, provided you are obtaining most of your calories from unprocessed whole plant foods, whilst minimising or avoiding meat and processed foods[3].

The other aspect of this confusion comes when people with insulin resistance, an inability to handle sugar in a normal way, eat fruit containing high amounts of fructose and then get a spike in their blood glucose levels. This does not mean that eating the fruit, such as a banana, is bad for you, only that your body is not handling the sugar correctly. To avoid the banana is like putting a sticking plaster over the problem rather than addressing the root cause. Insulin resistance, the underlying cause of type 2 diabetes, is due to accumulation of fat in the cells of the liver, muscle and pancreas such that insulin can no longer function as it should[4, 5]. This is caused by eating a diet high in animal-derived and/or processed foods, that deadly combination of saturated fat and free sugars. In fact, when eating the wrong types of food, you can accumulate fat inside muscle and liver cells even if you are of normal body weight; sometimes called TOFI – 'thin on the outside, fat on the inside'[6]. Eliminating these unhealthy foods from your diet can have an immediate effect on insulin resistance and within a few weeks eating fruit will no longer cause glucose levels to spike in your blood. In fact, randomised studies have shown that a low-fat vegan diet, high in fruit and vegetables, can reduce insulin resistance by reducing the amount of fat inside the cells and can be an effective treatment for patients with type 2 diabetes[7, 8].

Virtually every study that has looked at this question has found that those eating the most fruit (and vegetables) have the lowest risk of developing type 2 diabetes[9]. Researchers have even measured certain markers of fruit and vegetable consumption in the blood and found the higher the level of vitamin C and carotenoids, the lower the risk of developing type 2 diabetes[10]. A randomised study limiting fruit consumption in people with type 2 diabetes found no benefit for diabetes control and led the researchers to conclude that: 'The intake of fruit should not be restricted in patients with type 2 diabetes.'[11] People with type 2 diabetes who consume fruit regularly actually have a reduced risk of diabetic complications and a reduced risk of death[12].

Of course, a vegan or plant-based diet does not guarantee a life free of type 2 diabetes, or any disease for that matter, but it puts you in a pretty good position for maintaining optimal health. When compared with a conventional omnivorous diet, a plant-based diet, be it vegetarian or vegan, is associated with some of the lowest rates of type 2 diabetes[12, 13]. In addition, a low-fat vegan diet has been shown to be an effective treatment for type 2 diabetes, allowing a significant proportion of people to reduce or even come off their medications (achieving re-mission)[8], and is effective in treating both physical and mental health complications of the disease and improving quality of life[14]. These data are so compelling that the American College of Lifestyle Medicine has endorsed a plant-based diet as the preferred dietary approach for putting type 2 diabetes into remission[15].

The exciting news is that early signs suggest a 100% plant-based diet may even benefit people with type 1 diabetes, which is caused by an autoimmune destruction of the pancreatic cells such that the body no longer produces insulin. Although patients require life-long insulin replacement, the amount of insulin required to control blood glucose levels can vary based on diet and the associated level of insulin resistance. Insulin resistance can arise in people with type 1 diabetes for the same reason as those with type 2 diabetes: accumulation of fat inside the cells[16, 17]. Case studies suggest that a plant-based diet that includes the liberal consumption of fruit can reduce insulin resistance, thus leading to a reduction in insulin dose and improvement in cardiovascular risk factors[18].

6.3 If I have kidney problems, do I need to worry about the high potassium levels in fruit and vegetables?

The conventional teaching for patients with severe kidney disease, including those on dialysis, has been to restrict the consumption of foods high in potassium. That usually means restricting the intake of certain fruit and vegetables. This is because the kidneys struggle to eliminate potassium when they are not functioning well and hence patients invariably end up limiting the consumption of fruit and vegetables. This often leads to a deterioration in the quality of their diet and hence an increased risk of complications such as high blood pressure, high cholesterol and CVD. More recently, this thinking has shifted with health professionals and patient advocacy organisations, such as the National Kidney Foundation in the US, now actively promoting plant-based diets, rich in fruit and vegetables. The science has evolved, and studies have demonstrated that the potassium level in the food consumed does not always impact blood potassium levels in the body as the overall quality of the diet is probably more important[19].

In contrast to animal-based foods, plant foods, particularly fruit and vegetables, have an alkaline, rather than acidic, effect in the body. This helps facilitate the movement of potassium into the cells rather than remaining in the blood. In addition, not all the potassium from plant foods is absorbed and the high fibre content promotes excretion of potassium in the faeces. Having said this, caution may still be needed when consuming fruit juices, vegetables sauces and dried fruit[20].

Due to the alkalising effect of fruit and vegetable consumption, randomised studies have been conducted to investigate whether fruit and vegetables can be used as a treatment for patients with metabolic acidosis – that is, when the acid level in the blood is too high due to the inability of the kidneys to remove it. The conventional treatment is sodium bicarbonate tablets. When put to the test, fruit and vegetables performed just as well as sodium bicarbonate without causing high potassium levels and also resulted in improved cardiovascular health and lower medication costs[21]. In fact, a vegan diet has been shown to delay the need for dialysis in patients with end-stage kidney failure. In one patient included in the study, dialysis was delayed for nearly five years[22]!

Overall, there is emerging evidence that a plant-based diet may reduce the need for some kidney-protecting medications, reduce complications and favourably affect the progression of disease and even survival of those suffering from chronic kidney conditions[23]. Having said this, anyone with kidney failure should work together with a specialist dietitian and other members of their renal healthcare team when making changes to their diet.

6.4 Do I have to buy organic fruit and vegetables?

There are ongoing health concerns about ingesting pesticide and herbicide residues when consuming conventionally grown fruit and vegetables. In 2015, the International Agency for Research on Cancer (IARC) classified certain chemicals used in farming, including malathion, glyphosate and diazinon, as group 2 carcinogens, which means they *probably* cause cancer[24]. However, this has not been endorsed by regulatory authorities such as the European Food Safety Authority or the United Nations Food and Agriculture Organization (FAO). If applying the precautionary principle, it is then attractive to purchase organically grown fruit and vegetables as the application of synthetic chemicals is thereby avoided. This potentially applies to all foods, not just fruit and vegetables.

There are two main studies to date that have examined the impact of consuming organically produced foods, both animal and plant-derived, compared with those grown conventionally, on the risk of cancer. The first to be reported was from the Million Women study in the UK. This study included 623,080 middle-aged women who reported their consumption of organic foods and were followed for the next nine years. The results showed that organic food consumption was not associated with a lower risk of cancer in general but was associated with a 21% lower risk of non-Hodgkin lymphoma, a cancer of the lymphatic system[25]. The second study was from France and included 68,946 men and women followed for 4.5 years. This did demonstrate a significantly lower level of cancer, with a 25% reduction in those consuming the most organic foods. This was mainly due to a 76% reduction in risk for lymphoma and 34% reduction in the risk of post-menopausal breast cancer[26].

While these studies are thought-provoking, they report only an association rather than proving a causal relationship. Nonetheless, the association with lymphoma is indeed plausible given the higher risk of lymphoma in people who work on farms or live near large farms that spray high quantities of these chemicals[27]. In fact, settlement agreements have been reached for 100,000 lawsuits in the US involving claimants who have developed non-Hodgkin lymphoma after exposure to glyphosate, the herbicide in Roundup.

The current guideline for cancer prevention from the American Cancer Society acknowledges the possible link between chemicals used in farming and the development of cancer. Nonetheless, we must recognise that for most people organic food is neither accessible nor affordable. We therefore support the recommendations from the guidelines which state that consuming plenty of fruit and vegetables is a greater priority for human health than choosing organic produce[28].

We can also minimise our exposure to contaminants by choosing more fruit and vegetables from the 'Clean Fifteen' list and choosing organic versions of those on the 'Dirty Dozen' list. These lists updated annually, compiled by the Environmental Working Group, rank the pesticide contamination of 47 popular fruit and vegetables, most relevant for North America[29].

6.5 But my children won't eat fruit and vegetables?

We are not going to pretend to be experts in childhood nutrition. The key to encouraging the consumption of fruit and vegetables is to keep trying with a wide variety of options but without forcing. There will be fruits and vegetables that your children like more than others, which is fine. Research shows that children need to be offered a new food up to 20 times before it is accepted, so never give up[30].

Healthy habits should be fostered early in life as they will be the foundation for a healthy eating pattern in later life. Children raised vegetarian or vegan consistently eat more portions of fruit and vegetables a day than those eating an omnivorous diet[31]. In the UK, only 18% of children manage to consume five portions of fruit and vegetables a day and in Canada it's less than a third. These are rather dismal statistics. All families need to be prioritising fruit and vegetable consumption. Some strategies include using fruit and vegetables as snacks throughout the day and keeping them within easy reach in the fridge or dining table. Fruit and vegetables can be added into smoothies and sauces, which can increase the nutritional value of meals and snacks – for example, blending spinach into a tomato sauce or adding kale to a fruit smoothie. Eating meals together as a family has been shown to result in less fussy eating and improve the quality of a child's diet[32]. Role modelling is very effective, so be sure to practise what you preach, and your children will soon join you.

6.6 So which fruit and vegetables are the healthiest?

The key to a healthy diet is eating a wide variety of fruit and vegetables. As mentioned previously, in the American Gut Project, the healthiest gut microbiome was associated with the consumption of 30 different plant foods a week[33]. However, there are still some superstars amongst fruit and vegetables that should be prioritised in the diet. A good rule of thumb is that the darker the colour, the healthier the fruit or vegetable as this dark colour represents a greater concentration of antioxidants. Choosing red onion rather than white onion or an orange sweet potato rather than a plain white potato can elevate the nutritional content of your meal.

I've heard berries are particularly good?

When it comes to fruit, berries win the prize. Despite their small size, they really do pack a punch. Berries are a particularly concentrated source of antioxidants, powerful compounds that help to reduce oxidative stress and inflammation in the body[34]. Regular berry consumption has been shown to have a beneficial impact on cardiovascular risk factors including lowering blood levels of total cholesterol, LDL-cholesterol, triglycerides and glucose, and reducing blood pressure[34, 35]. The high flavonoid content of berries has been associated with protection against dementia[36, 37]. Flavanoids are a diverse group of naturally occurring compounds found in plants, associated with many health promoting effects, including antioxidant and anti-inflammatory properties. Berries may even have a role to play in the prevention and management of type 2 diabetes, with some studies demonstrating their ability to lower blood glucose and insulin levels and improve insulin sensitivity[39]. Berries are high in fibre yet relatively low in carbohydrates so are even championed by those on a low-carbohydrate diet.

And the cabbage family?

For vegetables, there are a few that should be incorporated daily or almost daily. Cruciferous vegetables, of the *Brassicaceae* family and whose flowers are shaped like a cross, come out top. This family of vegetables includes kale, broccoli, cauliflower, cabbage, Brussels sprouts and bok choy, which are rich in nutrients such as carotenoids, vitamins C, E, K and folate (vitamin B9). They seem to reduce the risk of virtually every illness you can think of. There are particularly strong associations with the consumption of cruciferous vegetables and a reduction in the risk of cancer. This is thought to be predominantly due to the sulphur-containing compounds called glucosinolates, which through the cooking, chewing and digestion process, are converted into several other compounds that benefit health. Two of these compounds, indole-3-carbinol and sulphoraphane, have been shown to have anti-cancer properties[40]. These compounds seem to act at a cellular level and even affect the expression of cancer genes. Laboratory studies have shown that these compounds can reduce inflammation and oxidative stress, differentially induce cancer cell death whilst preserving the function of normal cells and also switch on cancer-suppressor genes and switch off cancer-promoting genes[41].

What about vegetables that are high in nitrates?

Nitrate-rich vegetables, including leafy greens such as Chinese cabbage, rocket, pak choi, swiss chard and spinach, are an excellent daily choice[42]. These vegetables acquire nitrates from the soil in which they are grown. Interestingly, the nitrate content of organically grown produce will be lower as these farming systems do not use synthetic nitrate fertilisers. As we chew these vegetables, the nitrates are reduced to nitrites by the bacteria in our mouth and then these nitrites are available to be converted into nitric oxide. Nitrates are also directly absorbed in the small intestine. Nitric oxide is essential for maintaining the health of our blood vessels, keeping them dilated so blood can effectively reach our body organs, preventing blood cells sticking to the lining of the vessels and preventing platelets, involved in blood clotting, from aggregating[43]. Nitrate medications are in fact used in people with angina.

Beetroot is also a great source of nitrates and a randomised study of beetroot juice showed that its consumption could lead to a reduction in blood pressure to the same magnitude as medication[44]. Dr Caldwell B Esselstyn insists that patients in his prevent-and-reverse heart disease programme chew nitrate-rich greens as a snack six times a day to restore the health of their heart vessels[45]. With a dash of acetic acid from balsamic or other vinegar, which enhances the activity of the enzyme nitric oxide synthetase, the production of nitric oxide is further increased[46].

There is always confusion about why nitrates in vegetables are considered healthy whilst nitrates and nitrites in processed red meat pose a health risk. The higher protein content of meat and the lack of vitamins and other phytochemicals result in nitrates and nitrites being converted to nitrosamines, compounds that have been implicated in increasing the risk of bowel cancer. In contrast, the low protein content of nitrate-rich vegetables, and the abundance of antioxidants such as vitamin C, reduce the formation of nitrosamine and instead lead to the production of nitric oxide. Nitric oxide also has a crucial role to play in maintaining our immune system and defending us against infectious agents[47].

What about mushrooms and yeasts?

Mushrooms are high up on the list of must-eat foods, with several beneficial nutrients. They are a good source of fibre, high in protein (45% of calories), and are rich in phytochemicals (alkaloids, phenolic acids, flavonoids, carotenoids), selenium, vitamins (niacin, thiamine, riboflavin, vitamin C, folate and pantothenic acid and vitamin D if exposed to ultraviolet (UV) light from the sun or UV lamps) and important antioxidants ergothioneine and glutathione that are thought to play a significant part in the prevention of cancer. Mushrooms also contain beta-glucans, a type of fibre or polysaccharide carbohydrate, that are thought to be responsible for many of the beneficial properties, including lowering cholesterol, supporting the immune system and regulating blood glucose levels. They also have anti-cancer properties. Mushrooms may also exert beneficial health effects through their action as prebiotics, substances that induce the growth or action of our gut microbiota[47, 48].

A review of 17 observational studies concluded that when comparing those who ate the least mushrooms (less than once a week) with those who consumed the most (at least five times per week) there was a 44% reduction in the risk of cancer, with a reduction in breast cancer being most apparent[50]. In addition, a study of 15,546 participants from the US, with a median age of 44.3 years at baseline and followed for 19.5 years, showed that participants who reported eating mushrooms had a 16% reduction in risk of death compared with those who did not eat mushrooms at all. There was a dose-response, with the more mushrooms consumed the lower the risk of death. In this study, eating a serving of mushrooms per day instead of red or processed red meat reduced the risk of death by 35%[51].

Interestingly, in common with mushrooms, nutritional yeast, a commonly used condiment in a plant-based diet, is also a rich source of beta-glucans. It is a species of yeast known as *Saccharomyces cerevisiae*, which is grown specifically to be used as a food product. The yeast cells are killed during the manufacturing process, so this is not a live product. Studies have demonstrated nutritional yeast to have beneficial effects on the immune system[52].

And the onion family?

Finally in our top selection of vegetables are the allium family: onions, garlic, leeks and chives. They are high in beneficial sulphur compounds, which are responsible for their characteristic smell and taste. Studies have reported these vegetables to have a staggering array of health benefits ranging from anti-cancer to anti-inflammatory properties and benefits for cardiovascular health. For cancer, the strongest association is for a reduction in risk of gastric (stomach) cancer, and garlic and onions have also been associated with a reduced risk of oesophageal cancer. There may also be some benefit for the prevention of laryngeal cancer, prostate cancer and pre-cancerous polyps in the large bowel (colorectal adenomatous polyps).

Garlic has been shown in intervention studies to reduce

total and LDL-cholesterol and increase HDL-cholesterol levels. Garlic supplementation has been shown to reduce glucose levels in people with type 2 diabetes. It is also beneficial for reducing blood pressure and reducing the level of CRP (C-reactive protein), a marker of inflammation. Garlic and onions come out top in this family of vegetables, containing similar polyphenol and flavonoid compounds[53].

Conclusion

An acronym coined by Dr Joel Fuhrman is an excellent guide to the healthiest plant foods: G-BOMBS – Greens, Beans, Onions, Mushrooms, Berries, Seeds and nuts[54].

6.7 Should I do a juice fast now and again?

We came across juice fasting after watching the Netflix documentary *Fat, Sick and Nearly Dead*. The main subject of the documentary, Joe Cross, decided to reboot his health by drinking only fruit and vegetable juice for 60 days. During this time, he lost significant amounts of weight and reversed some aspects of his underlying autoimmune disease, managing to come off long-term medications. Along his journey, he meets a morbidly obese truck driver and helps him to regain his health through the power of juicing. There has also been a long history of using fruit and vegetable juicing as part of Gerson Therapy™, a whole-body approach for healing chronic disease, especially cancer[55]. To date, the evidence for any special healing power of juicing is limited and anecdotal at best. There are some case series of cancer patients benefiting from Gerson Therapy, but it is impossible to tease out what exactly may have benefited the patients in these reports as it is common for patients to have tried multiple different treatment approaches at the same time[56, 57].

Much of the perceived benefit of a juice fast comes from the associated fall in calorie intake and the removal of harmful foods such as ultra-processed and animal-derived foods. Any diet that reduces our calorie intake will result in weight loss and have beneficial knock-on effects of reducing blood lipids, blood pressure and inflammation and improving general metabolic health.

In fact, intermittent periods of fasting where calorie intake is drastically reduced for a short period of time, has been more extensively investigated and studies have shown benefits. Dr Valter Longo has brought his unique fasting-mimicking diet into clinical practice. This is a plant-based high-fat, low-calorie diet designed to mimic the effects of a total fast and used for five consecutive days per month. Calories are limited to around 1000 kcal on day 1 and then 800 kcal on days 2-5. In randomised studies he has shown that this type of short period of fasting can significantly reduce body weight and fat, lower blood pressure and decrease blood lipid levels, markers of inflammation and IGF-1 levels, suggesting this could be an approach for improving long-term health outcomes[58]. Fasting and juicing appear to have beneficial effects on the gut microbiome, which may in part account for the reported benefits[58, 59].

Dr Longo has also reported the initial findings of a small randomised study of his fasting-mimicking diet in patients with breast cancer receiving chemotherapy[61]. The results are certainly compelling, with the intervention group showing improved cancer cell death whilst sparing normal cells. However, these data alone are insufficient as yet to recommend this approach in clinical practice, but we will certainly be avidly assessing the evidence in this area as it evolves.

Juicing fruit and vegetables provides the body with a boost of vitamins, minerals, soluble fibre and an array of phytochemicals that many of us don't consume enough of, such as carotenoids, polyphenols and nitrates. Polyphenols are compounds with beneficial properties such as antioxidant, immunomodulatory and antimicrobial, and are also utilised by the gut bacteria. Juicing nitrate-rich vegetables has been shown to increase blood levels of nitric oxide, which we know to be beneficial for the health of our blood vessels[59]. Studies of adding vegetable juices to the usual diet have been reported to have benefits, including kale juice for reducing cholesterol levels[62], beetroot juice for reducing blood pressure[63], and carrot juice for reducing oxidative stress in survivors of breast cancer[64].

Can there be a downside?

It is important to distinguish juicing fresh fruit and vegetables from the consumption of store-bought fruit juices or sugar-sweetened beverages. In contrast to short duration use of fruit and vegetable juicing, longer term regular consumption of fruit juice may have adverse effects on health due to the free sugar content in the form of fructose and the lack of insoluble fibre. Several studies have now shown that fruit juice consumption may increase the risk of overweight and obesity, CVD, type 2 diabetes and cancer, and in children there is concern about an increased risk of tooth decay[64, 65]. A causal relationship cannot be demonstrated for certain, and it may be that people consuming the most fruit juice are also consuming fewer whole plant foods and more sugary foods and drinks in general.

The question then is whether a juice fast, or any sort of fast, is better than just consuming a whole food plant-based diet full of a variety of healthy plant foods. For us, the most compelling data presented to date come from Dr Valter Longo and his fasting-mimicking diet. However, until and when the global population adopt a healthy plant-based diet we will not know whether additional periods of fasting, be it with a meal replacement or juicing, add any advantages.

We should also acknowledge that fasting has been a part

of several cultures and traditions since time immemorial and so in and of itself is not a new concept. The science of how to incorporate it into our modern lives to support health and prevent chronic illness is still evolving.

Chapter 7

Eating whole grains

7.1 Why do I need to eat whole grains rather than refined grains?

A whole grain is one that is intact with all its layers. There are three layers to a whole grain: the bran (the outer, fibre-rich layer), the endosperm (the middle layer) and the germ (the inner nutrient-dense core). A refined 'white' grain, such as white rice or white flour, has had the bran and germ layer removed and hence lost most of the fibre, vitamins and minerals and phytochemicals. Refined grains such as wheat often have nutrients added back in to improve the nutritional value.

The terms 'cereal' and 'grain' are used rather interchangeably. A cereal is any grass cultivated for the edible components of its grain. A grain is the edible seed of a cereal grass. Examples of cereal grains include wheat, rice, oats, barley, rye, barley, millet, corn, triticale, and sorghum.

There is an abundant literature supporting the benefit of whole grain consumption for reducing the risk of many chronic diseases. Some of the strongest evidence is for colorectal cancer where studies have shown that consuming three portions of whole grains a day (90 grams) can reduce the risk by up to 20%[1]. It is likely that it is not only the fibre in whole grains that is responsible for this effect, but the intact whole grain itself. One of the largest studies to examine this question followed 478,994 adults from the US for 16 years. It showed that whole grain consumption, but not dietary fibre per se, reduced the risk of colorectal cancer by 24%[2]. This is because whole grains are more than just fibre and contain several other beneficial nutrients, including folate and other B vitamins, minerals, phenols, antioxidants and phytoestrogens.

Whole grain consumption has also been associated with a 32% reduction in the risk of type 2 diabetes[3], around a 20% reduction in the risk of cardiovascular diseases (CVD – heart disease and stroke)[4, 5] and a 17% reduction in the risk of dying from any cause[4]. Randomised studies have confirmed the benefit of whole grain consumption for reducing cardiovascular risk factors, including lowering high blood pressure, blood cholesterol and LDL-cholesterol, triglycerides, HbA1c (a marker of glucose control) and CRP (C-reactive protein), a marker of inflammation[6]. These benefits are seen with the consumption of three portions of whole grains a day (90 grams), with a portion being two slices of bread and one bowl of cereal, or one and a half pieces of pita bread made from whole grains. Benefits are seen with a wide variety of grains.

The same health benefits are not apparent for the consumption of refined grains. In addition to the loss of valuable nutrients, refined grains, such as white flour and white rice, are easily digested and absorbed, leading to a rapid and larger spike in blood glucose and insulin levels after a meal, an effect associated with worse health[7, 8, 9]. Although recent studies have shown that individuals can have different glucose responses to the same foods, most likely due to differences in their gut microbiome, there are some generalisations we can make[10].

The 'glycaemic index' of a food is a measure of how much it raises blood glucose levels compared with pure glucose. The 'glycaemic load' also takes into account the quality and quantity of the carbohydrate in the food and not just the amount so is probably a better reflection of the healthiness of a food. A diet composed of lower glycaemic foods is associated with a lower risk of heart disease, type 2 diabetes and overweight/obesity[9, 11]. In general, refined grains have a higher glycaemic index and load. White bread, for example, has one of the highest glycaemic effects of any food and is often used as the reference value by which to compare other foods[12, 13].

Having said all this, it's probably not worth getting too bogged down in comparing the glycaemic effect of different foods as things are not always straightforward. Different varieties of the same food can have a different glycaemic index. This is particularly relevant to rice[13]. Some of the adverse health outcomes associated with refined grains are in part due to the type of foods they are often found in, like cakes and pastries, which common sense tells us are not healthy.

For South Asians, carbohydrates often comprise 70–80% of the diet and up until recently carbohydrate sources such as rice were much less processed. Now, white, polished rice forms a large proportion of South Asian and other traditional diets, and this white rice has lost much of its fibre and nutrients. Several studies suggest that a diet heavily reliant on white rice can have adverse health outcomes. For example, a report from the PURE study (section 2.2), including 132,373 individuals from 21 countries, examined the impact of white rice consumption on the risk of type 2 diabetes. The results showed that those consuming the most white rice (more than 450 grams per day where 150 grams is 1 cup of cooked rice) had a 20% increased risk of developing diabetes compared with those consuming the least (less than 150 grams per day) and this association was particularly strong in people from South Asia, who had a 61% increased risk. The potential reasons for this are: the high glycaemic index and load of polished white rice, similar to eating white bread; the lower fibre intake; and also a possible contribution of the arsenic content in rice (although this had not been proven – see section 7.3)[14].

The weight of evidence supports eating whole grains over refined grains for their greater nutritional content, including fibre, and their lower glycaemic effect.

7.2 Should I avoid gluten?

The topic of gluten and its impact on health has become rather confused in the popular and medical literature. Most supermarkets and food outlets highlight their gluten-free products to consumers, a multibillion-dollar food trend. So, what is the truth behind gluten and its health impact?

Gluten is a family of proteins known as prolamins (primarily glutenin and gliadin) that is part of the protein in the endosperm of many cereal grains, such as wheat, barley and rye. Each type of cereal grain contains different amounts of gluten.

Coeliac disease is an autoimmune condition whereby the body's immune system reacts adversely to gluten, specifically gliadin. This abnormal immune response inadvertently attacks the small bowel leading to a number of symptoms and problems with nutrient absorption. The incidence of coeliac disease is around 1% in Europe and North America, with an increased risk in family members. Removal of gluten from the diet is a very effective treatment.

An even less common condition that requires avoidance of gluten is gluten ataxia in which the abnormal immune response to gluten damages the cerebellum (back part of the brain)[15].

Another 1% of the population may have a true allergy to wheat, and thus wheat consumption alone, rather than gluten, should be avoided[16].

There is a further group of individuals who may be classified as having a gluten-sensitivity, with symptoms of irritable bowel syndrome, who do not have coeliac disease or wheat allergy but show improvement in their symptoms after removal of gluten from their diet. This is now being termed 'non-coeliac gluten sensitivity', a diagnosis that can be challenging to make and has a reported prevalence of between 0.5 and 13% of the general population[17]. The evidence supporting the removal of gluten from the diet of individuals with symptoms of irritable bowel syndrome remains weak[18]. It may in fact be the fructan in wheat, a type of 'long chain sugar' that is the real culprit in individuals who respond to removal of wheat from the diet[19].

Many consider a gluten-free diet as a healthy option, when actually this approach can reduce the quality of the diet. It is worth noting that removing gluten from the diet also removes foods such as pastries, doughnuts and white bread, which is why some people notice immediate improvements to health. A study comparing the quality of a gluten-free diet with a gluten-containing diet found that gluten-free diets were more likely to be lower in dietary fibre, folate, protein, vitamin E, magnesium and potassium[20]. Other studies have found inadequate intakes of iron, zinc and calcium, higher intakes of saturated and hydrogenated fatty acids and higher glycaemic index and load of the diet[21]. Studies that have compared gluten-free supermarket products with similar gluten-containing ones have not been able to show a nutritional advantage, whereas some of the products can be lower in protein (which may not in itself pose a health problem) and fibre[22, 23]. In addition, these products can be significantly more expensive than their gluten-containing equivalents, with gluten-free breads, for example, being 400% pricier[24].

Given the robust evidence for including whole grains in the diet, limiting this important food group to avoid gluten can increase the risk of certain chronic diseases. A review of 27 studies found that a gluten-free diet led to a significant increase in total cholesterol, fasting glucose and body mass index (albeit still in the normal range)[25]. Although the overall impact on development of CVD remains uncertain, there are some concerns that the reduced consumption of whole grains in the context of a gluten-free diet may increase the risk of coronary heart disease, with those including gluten-containing whole grains in the diet reducing their risk of heart disease by 15%[26].

A review of 14 studies on patients with coeliac disease showed that those on a gluten-free diet had increased likelihood of non-alcoholic fatty liver disease and weight gain, a worse lipid profile and high blood glucose levels. Although the cause for this cannot be established for certain, it is thought that the inferior nutritional quality of a gluten-free diet may play a part[27]. Rapid and measurable changes become apparent in the composition of the gut microbiome within weeks of adopting a gluten-free diet, although the impact of these changes on overall health is yet to be determined[28]. Having said this, for those who do have to avoid gluten in their diet, eating more gluten-free 'pseudograins' such as amaranth, buckwheat, quinoa and millet is a good way to ensure a high-quality diet.

What about a link with dementia?

Despite the claims made in some popular books, there is little evidence to implicate gluten in the epidemic of dementia. A report from the Nurses' Health Study (section 1.4), specifically examined the impact of gluten consumption on brain health and cognitive function of 13,494 women with a median age of 60 years[29]. Long-term gluten consumption was not found to adversely affect cognitive function. In addition, short-term changes in gluten consumption did not impact cognitive function. The authors concluded: 'Our findings suggest that restricting dietary gluten for the purpose of maintaining or improving cognition is not warranted in the absence of coeliac disease or established gluten sensitivity.'

Conclusion

Overall, from the evidence we have, there is little reason for removing gluten from your diet unless you have a medically diagnosed condition that would benefit from this. In fact, eating gluten-free can reduce the overall quality of the diet, increase the cost, and potentially increase the risk of certain chronic diseases.

7.3 Brown rice contains arsenic so should I avoid this?

Rice is a major source of arsenic in the diet. The reason for this is that rice farming uses a lot of water when grown in flooded rice paddies and this water in many of the areas of the world responsible for rice production is contaminated with arsenic. Other foods that also have high levels of arsenic include seafood, mushrooms, poultry and even fruit juices. Arsenic in food and water has been implicated in an increased risk of cancer[30] and possibly CVD[31].

The reason rice is of particular concern is because it is a staple food for such a large proportion of the world and is also a staple for children. Whereas arsenic in water is regulated, arsenic in food is less so and, although there are recommendations for manufacturers, these are not legally enforced. There are farming methods for reducing arsenic in rice, including using less water rather than flooded paddies, an example being the System of Rice Intensification[32, 33]. In addition, cooking methods can help, so cooking rice in excess water, in the same way as pasta, and then draining this water, will significantly reduce the arsenic levels.

White rice contains less arsenic than brown, but we should be emphasising whole grains in the diet. So, our advice would be to mix up your whole grains and aim for a variety, including quinoa, couscous, bulgur, rye, barley, buckwheat and oats. Brown basmati from California, India, or Pakistan is the best choice as it has about a third less inorganic arsenic than other brown rice[34].

7.4 Are all whole grains healthy or are some better than others?

Overall, all whole grains are healthy and contain valuable nutrients. Eating a variety of grains will help you get the best out of the different quantities of nutrients in various grains. Nonetheless, as with all foods, you can optimise your choice by taking into account a few additional factors. The go-to person on this topic is Brenda Davis RD, acclaimed vegan dietitian, author of some of the most definitive books on vegan nutrition[35]. She makes some excellent and relevant observations:

- As with fruit and vegetables, the darker the grains the higher the amounts of antioxidants and phytonutrients. So black rice is healthier than brown and red quinoa healthier than beige.

- Different grains undergo various amounts of processing. The least processed the better, of course, as the processing reduces the nutritional value and increases the glycaemic index. Consequently, the best choices are intact whole grains such as barley, kamut, spelt, quinoa, rice and buckwheat. The next best choices are cut grains, such as steel-cut oats or bulgur. Rolled and shredded grains come next. Ground grains, which are essentially all flour products, should be eaten less frequently. Flaked and puffed grains are even more heavily processed and the least healthy choice.

- Bread has become a staple in many diets but given it is made of flour it is not the healthiest choice, with many commercial breads having added salt and sugar. It is preferable to make your own bread from whole grain flour or shop for such breads, although they are increasingly hard to find and often expensive. Bread made from sprouted whole grains also increases the nutritional value.

Another important issue to consider is the benefit of diversifying our diet and eating a wider range of plant foods including grains. It is incredible to think that just three grains, maize (corn), wheat and rice, make up 60% of the world's food energy intake[36], yet, the world has over 50,000 edible plants. Our diet has become so monotonous that globally, 75% of food is derived from 12 plant and five animal species. This dietary monotony is in part driven by our 'modern', industrialised agricultural system which is heavily reliant on monoculture farming. This in turn is contributing to a dramatic loss of plant diversity in our agricultural systems and threatens the resilience of our food system. Monoculture farming is also a major contributor to the degradation of soil health, leading to more widespread use of synthetic fertilisers and pesticides, which then results in loss of wildlife species and crucial soil organisms. Increasing the diversity of our diet will therefore not only improve the nutritional quality but also benefit the environment[37].

7.5 So why do some doctors recommend cutting carbs and grains for weight loss?

Low-carbohydrate diets and very-low-carbohydrate diets (including ketogenic diets) have traditionally been used for weight loss, and more recently for diabetes and other cardiometabolic risk factors such as hypertension and dyslipidaemia. Definitions vary in the literature. In the 2019 National Lipid Association review, a carbohydrate-restricted diet is defined as carbohydrate intake below the lower boundary of the acceptable macronutrient distribution range for healthy adults, which is considered to be 45-65% of total daily energy (TDE). A moderate-carbohydrate diet is defined as 26-44% TDE from carbohydrate (130-225 grams per day for a reference 2000 calorie daily diet), a low-carbohydrate diet as 10-25% TDE (50-130 grams per day), and a very-low-carbohydrate diet as 10% TDE (50 grams per day).

The current popular very-low-carbohydrate diet is the ketogenic diet which restricts carbohydrate to 20 to 50 grams per day, which is about 5 to 10% of TDE, with 70 to 80% of TDE from fat. Also of note is that the carbohydrate amounts relate to net carbohydrate, which is the grams of carbohydrate minus the grams of total fibre, which is also a carbohydrate but is not absorbed.

As discussed in Chapter 6, carbohydrates should not be considered as a food group and not all carbohydrate-containing foods are unhealthy. In fact, the healthiest foods on this planet are predominantly composed of carbohydrates: fruit, vegetables, whole grains and beans. The trouble is that in most high-income countries, and many others that are rapidly adopting the 'Western-diet pattern', most carbohydrates are consumed in the form of refined grains and free sugar, as part of processed and ultra-processed foods. In the UK, more than 50% of all foods bought in the supermarket are classified as ultra-processed[38] and in Canada the situation is similar[39]. On the surface of it, a low-carbohydrate diet that encourages people to give up refined sugar and grains will result in reduced calorie intake and weight loss. In fact, any diet that results in weight loss will have benefits for cardiovascular risk factors, such as high blood pressure, blood cholesterol and fasting glucose levels. For those with type 2 diabetes, the removal of refined carbohydrates will bring down blood sugar levels but unfortunately does not reverse the root cause, insulin resistance.

Unfortunately, excluding carbohydrates that come from whole plant foods, including whole grains, fruit and beans, is storing up longer term problems. Large prospective cohort studies confirm that low-carbohydrate diets increase the risk of CVD and death. A study published in the *European Heart Journal* in April 2019 examined the relationship between low-carbohydrate diets, all-cause death, and deaths from coronary heart disease, cerebrovascular disease (including stroke) and cancer in 24,825 participants in the US National Health and Nutrition Examination Survey (NHANES) during 1999 to 2010[40]. Compared with participants with the highest carbohydrate consumption, those with the lowest intake had a 32% higher risk of death from all causes over an average 6.4-year follow-up. In addition, risks of death from CVD, cerebrovascular disease and cancer were increased by 50%, 51% and 36%, respectively. In the same publication, researchers went on to confirm the results by performing a meta-analysis of nine prospective cohort studies (see section 1.4) with 462,934 participants and an average follow-up of 15.6 years. The results showed a 22%, 13%, and 8% increased risk in total, cardiovascular and cancer mortality with low- (compared with high-) carbohydrate diets. One of the lead authors, Professor Banach, has been quoted as saying: 'Low-carbohydrate diets might be useful in the short term to lose weight, lower blood pressure, and improve blood glucose control, but our study suggests that in the long-term they are linked with an increased risk of death from any cause, and deaths due to CVD, cerebrovascular disease, and cancer.'

A further paper from Dr Kevin Hall's team at the National Institute of Health has shed some light on why low-carbohydrate diets, high in fat, might have a detrimental effect on health[41]. He conducted a study on 17 participants who were admitted to a metabolic ward where all the food was provided, and detailed metabolic tests were performed. The study found that a ketogenic diet was associated with an increase in markers of inflammation and in LDL-cholesterol and did not improve insulin sensitivity or glucose regulation.

In 2019, the National Lipid Association reviewed the evidence for low-carbohydrate and very-low-carbohydrate diets (including ketogenic diets) for weight loss and cardio-metabolic risk factors and wrote a statement based on their findings[42]. They concluded that low-carbohydrate diets are not superior to other weight-loss diets and have no clear advantages for cardio-metabolic health.

There may be some short-term benefits (that is, for up to six months) but this type of diet is unlikely to be sustainable in the longer term. Some of the initial weight loss on a low-carbohydrate diet is due to water loss and there is concern about loss of lean muscle mass. Any short-term benefit for patients with diabetes has not been shown to translate into a longer-term benefit. The report highlights concern over the risk of adverse long-term health outcomes, including an increased risk of death. The report concludes by stating that patients should be encouraged to eat a diet composed of fruit, vegetables, whole grains, legumes, nuts and seeds due to consistent long-term benefits for health. This diet pattern can also be lower in carbohydrate if desired, with the help of a dietitian.

Similarly, the Scientific Advisory on Nutrition in the UK also published a review of low-carbohydrate diets for type 2 diabetes in 2021[43]. Overall, the recommendations are sensible and appropriately cautious. The report concluded that there are some short-term (up to six months) benefits for lower-carbohydrate diets on blood glucose regulation and triglyceride levels. They found no consistent evidence of reductions in body weight with lower-carbohydrate diets and no differences were observed between higher- and lower-carbohydrate diets on blood total cholesterol or LDL-cholesterol either in the shorter (three to six months) or longer ($\geq$12 months) term. The report acknowledges that the data reviewed relate only to Caucasians as there is very little information on low-carbohydrate diets in other ethnicities. The report also makes clear that those choosing a lower-carbohydrate diet should include whole-grain or higher-fibre foods and a variety of fruit and vegetables and limit their intake of saturated fats as per usual healthy-eating guidelines. The advice remains to consume 30 grams of fibre a day, which is very hard to do when cutting out healthy, carbohydrate-rich foods.

A further concern is that a low-carbohydrate diet centred

around animal-based foods may lead to progression of coronary heart disease[44]. An analysis from the CARDIA study (Coronary Artery Risk Development in Young Adults) investigated the impact of a low-carb diet on coronary artery calcium (CAC) scores in 2226 participants who were in their 40s at recruitment. CAC reflects the presence of atherosclerotic plaque in the coronary arteries and is associated with the risk of CVD. Diet was analysed and correlated with CAC scores determined by computed tomography at year 15 of follow-up and then at years 20–25 follow-up. The risk of progression of CAC was determined. The results showed an inverse relationship between carbohydrate intake and presence and progression of CAC scores. A higher carbohydrate intake was associated with a 15–25% reduction in risk of CAC progression. When analysing the components of the diet, the results showed that those consuming a low-carbohydrate diet, in which carbohydrates were replaced by animal protein and fat, had the greatest risk of CAC progression during the follow-up, with an increased risk of 45%. However, replacing carbohydrates with plant sources of fat and protein did not have an impact on CAC progression. These findings were despite the fact that the study did not elucidate the quality of carbohydrates consumed, refined versus complex. The authors of this paper concluded: 'Taken together, we found that low-carbohydrate diets beginning at early adulthood were associated with an increased risk of subsequent CAC progression in middle age, particularly when animal protein or fat ...are increased. As a popular strategy for weight management, long-term animal-based low-carbohydrate diets should be advocated with great caution to avoid its potential impact on coronary atherosclerosis.'

The reasoning behind the 'low-carb' approach for type 2 diabetes in particular is that if you limit the availability of sugar in the diet, then blood sugar will remain stable and there will be a reduced requirement for insulin. However, substituting carbohydrates with protein and fat, particularly if from animal sources, does not reduce insulin resistance beyond that achieved through weight loss. Therefore, if people with type 2 diabetes on a low-carbohydrate diet decide to eat a carbohydrate-rich food, such as a banana, their blood sugar will still become abnormally elevated because of the persisting insulin resistance. In contrast, a high-carbohydrate, high-fibre, plant-based diet in people with diabetes has been shown to reduce insulin requirements and, in some, reverse diabetes even without weight loss, thus demonstrating the power of whole plant foods to reverse insulin resistance[45].

If a low-carbohydrate approach is used, it may be prudent to do this in the context of a plant-based diet. The Eco-Atkins diet, pioneered by Dr David Jenkins, is a plant-based low-carbohydrate diet with increased protein and fat from gluten and soya products, nuts and vegetable oils. It may have an advantage for managing cardiovascular risk factors when compared with a low-fat approach[46].

Chapter 8

Eating beans and legumes

8.1 What is the difference between a bean and a legume?

The term 'legume' refers to any plant from the *Leguminosae* (or *Fabaceae*) family. *Leguminosae* are also collectively called the 'legume family'. It is the third largest family of flowering plants, consisting of 751 genera and about 20,000 species. A legume plant bears its 'seed', or 'grain', inside a pod (which is also called the fruit of the legume) and characterised by having compound, stipulate leaves. Legumes are notable in that they have symbiotic nitrogen-fixing bacteria, *Rhizobia*, in structures called root nodules. These bacteria have the special ability of fixing nitrogen from atmospheric, molecular nitrogen (N2) into ammonia (NH3) – that is, of drawing nitrogen out of the atmosphere and converting it into other nitrogen-containing compounds that the plants can readily use or put back into the soil to be used as a biological form of nitrogen.

Beans are one of the many types of legume. Similar to the term 'legume' that can pertain to the plant or its fruit (or seed), the term 'bean' can likewise refer to the plant or the seed. Different beans can come from different genera in the legume family – for example, the genus *Phaseolus*, consists of about 70 species and these are commonly called the 'wild bean plants'.

The term 'pulse' is reserved for legume crops harvested solely for the dry seed which has little or no oil content. The United Nations Food and Agriculture Organization recognises 11 types of pulses: dried beans, dried broad beans, dried peas, chickpeas, cow peas, pigeon peas, lentils, bambara beans, vetches, lupins and nes pulses. (Nes pulses are the minor pulses that don't fall into one of the other categories.) Other grain legumes, such as groundnuts (peanuts) and soya beans, have a high oil content and are referred to as oil seeds, not pulses.

When legume beans are harvested green in pods, they are considered as vegetables – for example, peas, French beans.

8.2 What is the issue with lectins in beans? Does this mean we shouldn't eat beans?

Most people had not heard or worried about lectins in food until the publication of the book called *The Plant Paradox: The Hidden Dangers in 'Healthy' Foods That Cause Disease and Weight Gain* by Dr Steven Gundry. The book tries to persuade readers that lectins in food are toxic, a key driver of our epidemic of chronic disease, and exposure should be minimised. The premise of this book is not at all supported by the science.

Lectins are a group of proteins that bind carbohydrates and are found in all plants as well as dairy, eggs, seafood and yeast. The highest amounts are found in raw beans and whole grains. There is no doubt that eating raw beans can be poisonous, particularly reported with consumption of raw kidney beans, which are high in a lectin known as phytohaemagglutinin that causes clumping of red cells and can also cause gastroenteritis[1].

Plants use lectins as a form of defence against predators such as insects and fungi[2]. The hypothesis put forward by Dr Gundry and his followers is that these proteins can bind to cells in the gut and cause 'leaky gut', leading to inflammatory disorders, including autoimmune diseases.

The truth is that no one eats raw beans and that lectins in whole grains and beans are inactivated within 15 minutes of cooking[3]. Lectins in some foods, such as tomatoes, lentils, chickpeas and peas, are not toxic at all. Common sense tells us that eating fruit, vegetables, whole grains and beans is healthy in spite of the lectin content. If proof is needed, we only need look again at the longest living and healthiest populations on this planet, found in the Blue Zones, and observe that whole grains and beans are staple components of these Blue Zone diets[4].

In fact, lectins have been associated with anti-cancer properties. Many lectins are resistant to digestion, passing through the cells of the gastrointestinal tract lining into the circulation. Studies have shown that these can bind preferentially to the surface of cancer cells and induce cancer cell death[5]. Mistletoe lectins have been the most extensively investigated for their anti-cancer properties and mistletoe is the most commonly prescribed complementary therapy in advanced cancer. Randomised studies have been conducted and some have demonstrated efficacy, including a study in patients with pancreatic cancer where treatment with mistletoe prolonged survival, albeit only by a median of two months[6].

Whenever you are told one nutrient or food is either the cause of all your health problems or has the potential to cure all your health problems, you can assume it is too good to be true. The health-promoting properties come as part of the whole food and the true impact of the whole food cannot be understood by studying only its individual components.

8.3 How do we know beans and legumes are so good for health?

Beans and other legumes are a key source of healthy nutrients, including fibre and the B vitamins (including folate, thiamine, riboflavin, niacin, pantothenic acid and B6), manganese, magnesium, copper, iron, potassium, zinc and phosphorus, to name a few. They are also an excellent source of protein, which comes in a much healthier package than animal protein, without cholesterol, saturated fat, haem iron or salt. One serving of cooked legumes (30-40 grams) can provide around 115 calories, 20 grams of carbohydrate, 7-9 grams of fibre, 8 grams of protein and 1 gram of fat. They also have a low glycaemic index[7]. Study after study has shown that choosing beans rather than meat, eggs, dairy or even fish improves health. For example, one of the most comprehensive reviews on the topic of animal versus plant protein showed that the consumption of plant protein instead of animal protein reduced the risk of dying by 8% and reduced the risk of dying from cardiovascular disease (CVD) by 12%. There was also a dose response relationship, with a 5% reduced risk of death for every 3% extra plant protein consumed[8].

Other studies have compared individual sources of protein. For example, a study of more than 400,000 men and women in the US who were followed for 16 years showed that just replacing 3% of protein from red meat, eggs and dairy with plant sources could reduce the risk of dying from any cause and from CVD by the order of 10-25%[9]. That is huge!

Eating beans instead of meat helps to maintain a healthy weight[10], reduces the risk of type 2 diabetes[11] and may even reduce the risk of some of our commonest cancers, including prostate and colorectal cancer[12, 13]. A randomised study of 121 people with type 2 diabetes showed that just adding one cup of legumes to their diet daily significantly improved blood glucose control, reducing HbA1c (haemoglobin A1c) levels and the coronary heart disease risk score, mainly due to a lowering of blood pressure but also lowering blood cholesterol and triglyceride levels[14]. That's a rather impressive result from just adding a single food.

Importantly, beans and legumes are one of the cheapest foods you can buy, providing more nutrients per calorie than any other food[15].

8.4 What about soya? Even though it's a legume I have heard it is bad for health?

The question of soy (North American term) or soya (European term) in the diet continues to cause confusion, even amongst health professionals. It is an example of how nutrition myths can continue to be propagated even if we have solid science proving otherwise. The bottom-line is that minimally processed soya foods, such as tofu, tempeh, miso, edamame and soya milk, are a healthy addition to any dietary pattern and especially a plant-based diet. Soya contains all nine essential amino acids, and soya protein has a biological value similar to meat protein[16]. It is also a good source of fibre, calcium and omega-3 fatty acids. Clinical studies have shown that the consumption of soya foods can have an array of health benefits. It is remarkable to consider how just one type of legume can have so many different beneficial effects and helps explain why it is a staple food in many traditional Asian diets.

A huge study incorporating all the best evidence we have to date showed that soya consumption has well-established benefits for reducing the risk of CVD, both stroke (18% reduction) and ischaemic heart disease (17%). This may be in part due to the ability of soya protein to lower cholesterol levels. In the case of cancer, there are benefits for reducing the risk of ovarian (48% reduction), prostate (29%), breast (13%), colorectal (21%), gastric (22% for non-fermented soya), lung (17%) and endometrial (19%) cancers. The only word of caution for cancer is an increased risk of gastric cancer (17%) in men consuming 1-5 cups of miso soup per day, likely due to the high salt content. The study also showed a benefit of soya consumption for perimenopausal symptoms in women, especially in relation to hot flashes. Other benefits reported included reduced risk of kidney disease, better cognitive function, reduced risk of type 2 diabetes, healthy weight and improved bone health in women. The only side effect of soya consumption reported in studies was gastrointestinal symptoms[17].

The misconceptions around soya come from the thinking that soya and the isoflavones (plant oestrogens) it contains can disrupt the human endocrine system – that is, the hormones of the body – and in doing so cause negative effects such as breast cancer, altered male and female hormones, reduced fertility and thyroid dysfunction (see the rest of this chapter for more detail on these questions). A review looking at all the data so far, including clinical studies, observational studies and systematic reviews and meta-analyses that examined the relationship between soya and/or isoflavone intake and related endpoints, concluded that there was no evidence that isoflavone intake affected thyroid function, female or male hormones or fertility, and isoflavones could not be classified as endocrine (hormone) disrupters[18].

Of course, a small proportion of people, no more than 0.5% of the population, are allergic to soya protein and therefore should avoid any foods that contain it[19].

A commonly cited concern is the genetic modification of soya crops and the associated requirement for herbicides and pesticides, with the potential negative consequences for the natural environment and human health. Whilst most soya produced worldwide is genetically modified, and used as a feed for food animals, it is not difficult to find soya that has not been genetically modified for our direct consumption.

8.5 Does soya increase the risk of breast cancer?

You may wonder why there is still doubt about the health

benefits of soya. As we said earlier in this chapter, it contains phyto-oestrogens (plant oestrogens) called isoflavones. These isoflavones can bind to oestrogen receptors. In some rodent studies, high doses of isoflavones have been shown to increase the risk of breast cancer[20]. Humans do not consume the high amounts of isoflavones used in these studies, nor are we rodents. The subject of animal research and its impact on human research is a topic for another book!

Humans have two types of oestrogen receptor: alpha and beta. Human oestrogen has a preference for alpha receptors, but phyto-oestrogens prefer binding to beta receptors. Depending on the tissue, phyto-oestrogens can either have a pro-oestrogenic effect or an anti-oestrogenic effect, thus soya is known as a 'selective oestrogen receptor modulator'[21]. In breast tissue, isoflavones in soya have an anti-oestrogen effect and there is no doubt that consumption of soya foods can help to reduce the risk of breast cancer in women, particularly if their consumption is started in childhood and adolescence[22]. For example, in one study regular consumption of tofu was shown to reduce the risk of breast cancer by around 22% when comparing those who ate the most versus those who ate the least. For every 10 grams per day consumed there was a 10% reduction in the risk of breast cancer[23].

In the Adventist Health Study-2 (section 1.4), swapping dairy milk for soya milk reduced the risk of breast cancer by up to 32%[24]. Soya consumption may also help reduce the risk of breast cancer recurrence in women who have been treated for that condition and improve survival. Interestingly, this applies to people who have had oestrogen receptor positive breast cancers as well as those with oestrogen negative breast cancers, suggesting that the phyto-oestrogen effect is not the whole story when it comes to the protective effects of soya[25].

Soya has different effects in different tissues. In bone, soya can have a pro-oestrogen effect and its consumption may help support bone health with ageing[26]. Soya consumption may also be useful at combating menopausal hot flashes, a pro-oestrogenic effect[27]. So, all in all, soya is a great addition to the diet and should be consumed regularly, aiming for two portions (160 grams) per day.

8.6 What about soya consumption in men? Does it have feminising effects?

Again, the concern here stems from the presence of plant oestro-gens and rare case reports where individuals have consumed huge amounts of soya – for example, a man who developed enlarged breasts and high blood oestrogen levels after drinking 3 litres of soya milk a day for a prolonged period[28]. The truth remains that multiple studies have shown that the regular consumption of sensible amounts of soya foods daily has no effect on male hormones, does not lead to enlarged breasts and has no impact on fertility. An updated, meta-analysis of 41 studies from 2021 showed that, regardless of the dose or length of study, neither soya protein nor isoflavones have any effect on levels of testosterone, oestrogen or sex hormone binding globulin in men[29]. If as a man you are worried about exposure to female hormones, then our best advice is to avoid dairy consumption. Milk produced from pregnant cows has been shown to increase oestrogen and progesterone levels in consumers and may even reduce testosterone levels in men[30, 31].

What about prostate cancer?

There is actually good evidence supporting soya consumption for prostate cancer prevention in men[32]. In fact, in the Adventist Health Study, men consuming soya milk at least once a day had a 70% reduction in the risk of prostate cancer[33]. If you already have a diagnosis of prostate cancer, adding soya to your diet could also help.

One study examined the impact of soya intake on prostate cancer progression. Men awaiting prostate surgery were randomly assigned to eating a diet that was either high in soya or was not. In the soya group there was a significant decrease in the PSA (prostate-specific antigen – a marker of prostate cancer growth) level when compared with the control group[34]. Another study treated men with prostate cancer with three servings of soya milk per day for 12 months and also showed a fall in PSA levels[35].

8.7 Does soya affect the thyroid gland?

There have previously been concerns that isoflavones in soya can adversely affect the function of the thyroid gland. However, there is no scientific evidence to support this claim in otherwise healthy children and adults as long as iodine intake is adequate[36, 37]. The only connection with thyroid health is in people who have an underactive thyroid gland and require thyroid hormone replacement. Soya, and other nutrients, can interfere with the absorption of these thyroid hormones and therefore its best to take thyroid hormone tablets on an empty stomach, such as half an hour before breakfast, and not within one hour of consuming soya-containing foods[38]. The main concern for thyroid health in any diet pattern is ensuring adequate intake of iodine, one of the commonest nutrient deficiencies globally[39].

8.8 But I have irritable bowel syndrome and beans make this worse?

Many people believe that they have irritable bowel syndrome (IBS), a collection of digestive symptoms including abdominal pain, bloating, gas and a change in bowel habit – either diarrhoea or constipation[40]. It appears to be an increasingly prevalent syndrome in Western countries, and many find they have certain dietary triggers. These can often be foods that are high in FODMAPs – fermentable oligosaccharides, disaccharides, monosaccharides and polyols – that resist digestion and are fermented by gut bacteria, producing gas[41]. Beans, legumes and pulses are often associated with excess gas and bloating, regardless of whether someone has IBS, due to their high FODMAP content and particularly the presence of galacto-oligosaccharides. The gas produced by the gut bacteria that digest these carbohydrates can get trapped and give the feeling of bloating and cause flatulence. A therapeutic low FODMAP diet may be a short-term solution for people with IBS, but in the longer term there are concerns that this type of diet overly restricts health-promoting foods, may adversely alter the gut microbiome and may affect the nutritional adequacy of the diet[42]. Some of these issues can be overcome with support from a dietitian or nutritionist.

Bloating and flatulence can be a particular problem when someone transitions from a standard meat-based Western diet to a plant-based diet as there is a sudden increase in their diet of these high-FODMAP foods, which also include fruit, whole grains and many common vegetables. People often report problems when beans are introduced into their diet and this is seen as a barrier to adopting a fully plant-based diet[43, 44].

There are several ways to try and reduce the impact on the digestive system:

- Start with small portions and with smaller-sized legumes, such as lentils, letting your gut adapt to the increase in fibre and oligosaccharides.
- Try various ways of significantly reducing the oligosaccharide content without reducing the nutritional value, including:
  - soaking dry beans and legumes overnight and

draining out the water before cooking and then cooking till very soft[45];

o   cooking in alkaline water by adding sodium bicarbonate[46];

o   germinating or sprouting, which actually increases the nutritional value and the digestibility of the protein[47];

o   cooking with carminatives – herbs and/or spices that reduce gas formation or help expel gas, including cumin, asafoetida, fennel, peppermint, turmeric, ginger and kombu, a Japanese seaweed[48].

In addition to all these measures, remember to eat slowly, chew well and drink plenty of water as you increase the fibre content of your meals.

Chapter 9

Eating nuts and seeds

9.1 Why should we be nuts about nuts?

Nut consumption came into prominence back in the early 1990s with the publication of two studies from Loma Linda University. The first was from the Adventist Health Study, which included 31,208 participants and showed that participants consuming nuts more than four times per week, when compared with those eating nuts less than once per week, had a 51% reduced risk of having a heart attack and a 48% reduction in risk of dying from heart disease[1]. The second, a small randomised study in 18 men who were assigned to either a standard healthy diet or one that included walnuts as 20% of energy (replacing fatty foods, meat and added fats) demonstrated a significant reduction in blood cholesterol levels in the walnut group[2].

Since then, the number of studies and publications on the impact of nut consumption has risen exponentially. The findings are exceedingly consistent, with the consumption of around 30 grams of nuts on most days of the week associated with a significant reduction in the risk of developing cardiovascular disease (CVD) and dying from it. The findings are most consistent across studies with regard to heart disease compared to stroke.

Interestingly, it may be that nut consumption has a greater impact on reducing the risk of death from heart disease rather than preventing its development in the first place. An analysis of 19 studies on the topic showed that eating nuts regularly reduced the risk of developing CVD by 15% and the risk of dying from CVD by 23%[3]. The greater impact on reducing death is hypothesised to be because nut consumption reduces the risk of arrhythmias (abnormal heart rhythm), a cause of sudden death. This sounds like a very similar story to that of fish consumption (section 5.1)!

Nut consumption has been associated with a significantly reduced risk of cancer, in the order of 15%[4], and of developing type 2 diabetes[5], although some of this benefit may be due to better weight control in regular nut consumers[6]. The more consistent finding in people with type 2 diabetes is a significant reduction in the risk of developing and dying from CVD[7].

Nut consumption may help us to live longer; one study calculated that an estimated 4.4 million premature deaths in the Americas, Europe, Southeast Asia and Western Pacific combined could be attributed to the fact that we are just not consuming enough[4]. Adding nuts to the diet even seems to improve sexual function in men[8].

We now understand some of the reasons for these beneficial effects. Nuts are powerhouses of healthy nutrients, including being an excellent source of protein, unsaturated fats, fibre, tocopherols (vitamin E family of compounds), folic acid, vitamin B6, calcium, magnesium, copper, zinc, selenium, phosphorus, arginine, potassium, niacin, phytosterols and polyphenols. The impact on heart health is partly due to the high content of unsaturated fatty acids, both monounsaturated and polyunsaturated, which act to reduce blood cholesterol and triglyceride levels[9]. Plant sterols also reduce blood cholesterol by preventing the absorption of dietary cholesterol in the gut[10]. Pistachios have the highest amount of phytosterols with almonds coming in second.

Arginine found in nuts can be used to make nitric oxide, which is required to dilate the blood vessels, and keep blood flowing to the vital organs. Nuts also improve the functioning of one of the most important cell types in the body, the endothelial cell. These cells line the inside of our blood vessels and it is the constant damage to this layer of cells that ultimately leads to atherosclerosis, the cause of heart attacks and most strokes[11, 12].

Nuts are useful for controlling blood sugar levels, especially regulating glucose levels after a meal, and reducing insulin resistance. They have been shown to be a useful addition to the diet in patients with type 2 diabetes[13, 14]. They are also known for their antioxidant ability due to being one of the richest sources of vitamin E compounds and also the source of a number of different polyphenol compounds[15]. Pecans come in top, closely followed by walnuts, when it comes to antioxidant activity. Brazil nuts are unique in having a high content of selenium, which also contributes to their antioxidant effects; one to two Brazil nuts per day provides us with the recommended daily intake of selenium[16].

9.2 Don't nuts make you put on weight?

The misguided low-fat marketing campaign back in the 1980s has mistakenly led us to believe that all fats are bad and contribute equally to poor health. This could not be further from the truth. Mono- and polyunsaturated fats, especially when replacing saturated fat in the diet, are associated with better health outcomes[17]. Given the higher calorie or energy density of fat (9 kcal/g versus only 4 kcal/g for protein and carbohydrate), it is also assumed that any high-fat food increases the risk of weight gain. Once again, this is not true and especially in relation to the consumption of nuts. Nuts are composed of at least 50% fat, with some nuts containing up to 80%. Despite this, incorporating them into your diet does not have an effect on body weight. In fact, nut consumption may be associated with a healthier body weight. How can this be?

A simple answer is that people regularly eating nuts are in general consuming a healthier diet. Nuts are likely to have been chosen instead of chocolate, crisps and/or cake, for example. There are also reasons that are intrinsic to the specific composition of nuts. Nuts are high in fibre with one serving providing somewhere between 2 and 3.5 grams of fibre depending on the nut, with almonds and peanuts topping the chart. Fibre delays gastric emptying, increasing the feeling of fullness or satiety, thus leading to reduced consumption of calories overall. The timing of nut consumption also has an impact here and eating them as a snack rather than as part of a meal has a greater effect on blunting hunger. Fibre can also bind fatty acids in the gut, leading to their excretion rather than absorption and thereby, to greater loss of calories in the faeces. In fact, not all the calories from the nuts are absorbed and studies have shown that somewhere in the region of 5-30% of calories are lost in the faeces depending on the nut.

Here the form of the nut is important too with greater fat absorption from nut butters than from the whole nut. In addition, the higher the fibre content of the overall diet, the lower the percentage of calories absorbed. Chewing nuts takes time and may lead to reduced food intake. Incomplete chewing of nuts could also contribute to the reduced absorption and increased faecal loss of fat. The high unsaturated fatty acid content is associated with both increased post-meal thermogenesis (heat generation) and resting energy expenditure. Unsaturated fatty acids also increase fatty acid oxidation, reducing body fat stores with, perhaps, a greater effect on visceral fat than subcutaneous fat, which may account for the benefits seen for metabolic health. The nutrients in nuts, particularly the fibre and polyphenols, also benefit gut health, although more research is needed in this area[18, 19, 20, 21].

9.3 If you were going to choose one type of nut to eat, which would be the best?

Our top pick has to be walnuts. It seems that just eating a single portion of walnuts a week can have a dramatic effect on cardiovascular health, with results from the Nurses' Health Study and the Health Professionals Follow-up Study reporting a 19% lower risk of CVD, a 21% lower risk of coronary heart disease (CHD), and a 17% lower risk of stroke[22]. This is likely to be due to the particularly high content of alpha-linolenic acid, an essential short chain omega-3 fatty acid, which has anti-inflammatory and anti-clotting effects as well as reducing triglyceride levels and the chances of developing an abnormal heart rhythm[23]. In the Nurses' Health Study, consuming two or more portions of walnuts per week reduced the risk of type 2 diabetes by 33%[24]. The largest and longest intervention study of walnuts in 634 older adults showed that regular consumption for two years reduced the levels of six out of 10 markers of inflammation in the blood, an effect that is not consistently seen with all nuts[25]. This study also demonstrated significant lowering of total and LDL-cholesterol in those consuming walnuts[26]. Randomised studies have also shown a beneficial effect on endothelial function[27].

Walnuts are high in antioxidant compounds, second only to pecans when tested in the laboratory[15]. They are particularly high in the vitamin E compound gamma-tocopherol, which is thought to be responsible for some of walnuts' unique anti-inflammatory and antioxidant properties. A small randomised study in patients with asthma showed that gamma-tocopherol supplements reduced markers of inflammation to a similar extent to inhaled steroids[28]. The antioxidant properties of walnuts may also be important in maintaining brain health with ageing, with some studies showing their ability to inhibit the formation of amyloid plaques, a key finding in Alzheimer dementia[29]. However, intervention studies have not been conclusive, with the largest and longest randomised study of walnuts mentioned above unable to show an overall benefit for brain health, although there may be a small benefit in those at higher risk of dementia[30].

Overall, walnuts make an excellent choice and a 30 gram portion per day will also provide you with sufficient amounts of the essential omega-3 fatty acid, alpha-linolenic acid mentioned above.

9.4 Should I avoid giving peanuts to my children in case they are allergic?

Parents often worry about nut allergy in children, and this frequently leads to avoidance of nut consumption. Peanut allergy is a particular concern and is the commonest food allergy in children, with a rising incidence. It affects one in 50 children in the UK and Canada. Of course, peanuts are not really a nut but a legume and grow on the ground, whereas other nuts are tree nuts.

Infants with severe eczema and/or egg allergy have a higher risk of peanut allergy[31]. However, rather than avoiding peanuts, which are a wonderfully nutrient-dense food for babies and children, the recommendations are to introduce peanuts early into the diet. Of note, whole peanuts should be avoided until after the age of 5 years to reduce the risk of choking, so here we are considering smooth nut butters and finely ground nuts.

A randomised study of 530 infants at high risk of peanut allergy due to having eczema or an egg allergy showed that early introduction of peanuts in the diet reduced the risk of allergy by 81%[32]. This led to a change in guidelines, which now recommend babies at high risk of peanut allergy have peanuts introduced into the diet between 4 and 6 months of age after allergy testing. Babies with mild or moderate eczema should have peanuts introduced (and maintained) into their diets around 6 months of age. Babies without eczema or any food allergy should have peanut-containing foods freely introduced into their diets at the time of weaning.

Despite these updated guidelines, a study from the US shows that paediatricians lack confidence in supporting the implementation of these recommendations and therefore parents with children at high risk of peanut allergy may not be well supported to introduce peanuts early in the diet[33].

9.5 What about eating seeds?

Officially, edible seeds include cereal grains, nuts, legumes, cocoa and coffee beans. Seeds are an embryonic plant enclosed in a protective outer layer and are part of the reproductive process in seed plants. Nuts are actually the seeds of plants. Here though we are referring to seeds from vegetables such as pumpkin, flowers such as sunflower or various crops like flax or hemp. These types of seed are full of healthy nutrients. They are an excellent source of protein, fibre and unsaturated fatty acids. They all have unique nutritional profiles. For example, pumpkin seeds are rich in iron, zinc, magnesium and one serving (30 grams) contains around 7 grams of protein. Sunflower seeds are rich in vitamin E, manganese and selenium. Sesame seeds are a great source of calcium, magnesium and zinc. Chia and flaxseeds are particularly high in fibre and a great source of essential omega-3 fatty acids. Chia seeds are also high in calcium.

For us, the mighty flaxseed probably comes out top for health-promoting benefits, although it's a tough choice. In addition to being a great source of fibre and omega-3 fats, they are high in lignans, a polyphenol with antioxidant and oestrogen-like properties[34]. A number of randomised studies have shown positive outcomes associated with their consumption. For example, a six-month study of 30 grams per day of flaxseeds was shown to significantly reduce both systolic and diastolic blood pressure by around 10 mm Hg and 7 mm Hg respectively, predominantly due to the action of alpha-linolenic acid[35, 36]. This effect is not dissimilar to that of prescription medications. A study of 10 grams of flaxseeds pre-mixed in cookies twice per day, versus placebo cookies, for 12 weeks in patients with type 2 diabetes showed significant reductions in body weight, fasting blood glucose and lipid levels[37].

Lignans in flaxseeds are converted in the gut to oestrogenic compounds and are hence known as phyto-oestrogens. These compounds have been shown to be beneficial for cancer prevention, in a similar way to the isoflavone phyto-oestrogens found in soya foods (section 8.4). A review of studies on breast cancer prevention concluded that 25 grams per day of flaxseeds may be associated with a reduced risk of developing breast cancer, may reduce the growth of breast tumours and could even improve survival in patients with breast cancer[38].

Similarly, there are benefits for prostate cancer in men. One study randomised 161 patients prior to surgery to 30 grams of flaxseeds per day versus a low-fat diet versus a low-fat diet plus flaxseeds and compared these with a control group. Results showed that those consuming flaxseeds had evidence of reduced cancer growth in the laboratory[39].

So, flaxseeds are an excellent addition to all diets, with a tablespoon a day or 30 grams being the right amount. In a 100% plant-based diet, this will also provide you with the required amount of essential omega-3 fatty acids. However, don't forget you need to eat ground or milled flaxseeds rather than whole to derive all the benefits.

9.6 Most of the studies showing nuts are healthy are sponsored by the nut industry, so can we really believe the data?

You are right to be sceptical. Vegans and plant-based doctors are quick to point out industry funding and conflicts of interest in meat, dairy and eggs studies, so examining funding sources of any food-related study is sensible. The reason is that industry-funded studies are more likely to show a positive outcome for their product than studies not funded by the relevant industry[40]. In part this is because the study design is often stacked in their favour, making the outcome a foregone conclusion. Unfortunately, it's very difficult to perform large, meaningful studies without the support of industry funders, which leaves us with a dilemma when it comes to studies on nut consumption. Many are indeed funded by the nut industry. The key is to be ready to spot a poorly designed study. For example, a study supported by the Almond Board of California compared almond consumption with pork consumption[41]. Well, it does not take a scientist to guess that almonds were going to come out top in this study.

Not all studies funded by industry are bad and one also needs to delve into the credibility of the researchers and make sure they work for institutions that are also independent and credible. Scientists are sadly not above being paid off to produce positive results from poorly designed studies[42, 43].

So, when it comes to studies of nuts, the best we can do is look at all the data in its entirety and check for consistency of results. Virtually all the thousands of studies conducted point to a positive benefit for health with no real downside, apart from to those people with a nut allergy. We have observational, laboratory, mechanistic and intervention studies that all consistently point towards benefits, which are then held up in meta-analyses, considered the most robust of analyses. Overall, this degree of consistency goes a long way to supporting the regular consumption of nuts.

Chapter 10

Foods and nutrients of special interest

10.1 Is it okay to use oil in food and cooking?

The advocates for a whole food plant-based diet are divided on the topic of added oils in the diet. The original adopters, including Dr T Colin Campbell and Dr Caldwell Esselstyn, recommend avoiding any added oils in the diet, including olive oil. However, consensus amongst the international cardiology community based on the scientific literature is that the addition of extra virgin olive oil (EVOO) is beneficial for heart health[1, 2]. This is because EVOO is high in monounsaturated fatty acids (mostly oleic acid), tocopherols (vitamin E compounds) and polyphenols. Studies show that replacing saturated fat (predominantly from animal sources) in the diet with monounsaturated fat from EVOO has a beneficial effect on blood lipid levels and consequently improves heart health[3]. The high polyphenol content contributes to counteracting oxidative stress[4]. In fact, the European Food Safety Authority allows for two health claims to be made to support the consumption of olive oil based on the properties of oleic acid and the polyphenols[5, 6]. When it comes to the polyphenols it states: 'Olive oil polyphenols contribute to the protection of blood lipids from oxidative stress. The claim may be used only for olive oil, containing at least 5 milligrams of hydroxytyrosol and its derivatives (e.g. oleuropein complex and tyrosol) per 20 grams of olive oil. In order to bear the claim, information shall be given to the consumer that the beneficial effect is obtained with a daily intake of 20 grams of olive oil.'

One common reason cited for avoiding EVOO is that in some small, isolated studies EVOO has been shown to impair flow-mediated vasodilatation (FMD), an indicator of endo-thelial function[7]. Impaired endothelial function is a major driver of atherosclerosis. However, a 2015 meta-analysis suggested that olive oil had a favourable effect on FMD[8]. Additionally, it is correctly argued that the polyphenol content is not all that remarkable when compared with whole plant foods. In a study that quantified the 100 richest sources of polyphenols and ranked them in order of the absolute content, EVOO ranked number 61 with a polyphenol content of 62 milligrams per 100 grams. In comparison, black olives ranked 19th and green olives 25th, with polyphenol contents of 569 milligrams per 100 grams and 346 milligrams per 100 grams, respectively. Blueberries ranked 20th with 560 milligrams per 100 grams, almost 10 times the content of olive oil. The top 10 foods included herbs and spices and dark chocolate[9].

There has never been a study of a whole-food plant-based diet with and without extra virgin olive oil. In fact, there are many healthy populations, including amongst the Blue Zones, who thrive on a low-fat diet that does not include EVOO. Examples are the indigenous South American Tsimane population[10] and Okinawans eating their traditional diet[11]. With 130 calories per tablespoon (17.7 millilitres), there needs to be a balance between this high-calorie density versus the nutritional benefits, especially since as a society we are facing an obesity crisis. Most people would use more than a tablespoon of olive oil for salad dressings or for cooking and hence the calorie content of the meal soon escalates. It should also be noted that the health benefits are mostly associated with the highest quality olive oil

– extra virgin – which is pressed from fresh olives, under cool temperatures, without the use of chemicals, hence preserving a higher polyphenol content. This comes with a price tag of course.

For very-high-temperature cooking, olive oil is less suitable than oils such as canola oil (often called rapeseed oil in the UK) and avocado oil, which have higher smoking points. Olive oil is fine for sautéing, for example, but not for deep frying, a cooking method probably best avoided anyway. There is similarly divided opinion on canola oil, partly because of the genetic modification of the canola plant. We won't be getting into the debate about GMOs, but suffice it to say that the end product, canola oil, does not contain DNA or proteins, just fat and a few vitamins. The scientific literature does confirm that canola oil is a healthy choice if you are going to use oil in your diet, as it is an oil that is high in monounsaturated fats and alpha-linolenic acid (ALA). A review of 42 clinical studies on the impact of canola oil on CVD risk factors found that canola oil improves blood lipid profiles, and to a greater degree than olive oil and sunflower oil[12].

This topic can get confusing when it need not be. Anxiety over added oil may lead to restricted eating patterns. Fats are, of course, an essential part of the diet and there is no right or wrong answer for how much should be included as long as they are derived from healthy plant sources. We leave you with our take home messages:

1. EVOO is a source of monounsaturated fatty acids and polyphenols and overall, the scientific literature supports its consumption for heart health.

2. EVOO, or any oil for that matter, is not essential in the diet, as unsaturated fats and polyphenols can easily be obtained from whole-plant sources.

3. Given the expense of high-quality oils you may prefer to use that money on buying more fruit and vegetables, which are essential components of the diet.

4. If you are young, fit, physically active, an ideal body

weight and free from health problems, then the addition of small amounts of EVOO and other oils, such as hemp seed, flaxseed/linseed, walnut and avocado oil to aid nutrient absorption and obtain essential fatty acids, is absolutely fine. It just comes down to personal preference.

5. We suggest that if you are trying to lose weight then adding calorie-dense oils to your diet, regardless of their health benefits, may make weight loss harder to achieve.

6. If you have established atherosclerosis, then the only diet shown to halt its progression is a no-oil whole-food plant-based diet as per the protocols used by Drs Esselstyn and Ornish. Certain inflammatory and autoimmune conditions also seem to be aggravated by the addition of processed oils to the diet, including lupus, rheumatoid arthritis, multiple sclerosis and polycystic ovarian syndrome (PCOS). In these situations, we would definitely recommend limiting added oil in the diet.

7. Finally, the most important take-home message is that it is always best to concentrate on the quality of the whole diet rather than individual components. A diet centred around whole plant foods, whether it contains EVOO or not, is the healthiest choice you can make.

10.2 Isn't coconut oil healthy?

Highly successful industry marketing has convinced many that coconut oil is a 'health food' with magical properties. Coconut oil is almost all fat, most of which is saturated fat. The predominant fat is lauric acid, with 25% composed of myristic and palmitic acids (also found in meat and dairy). Although not all saturated fats behave in the same way, all three, including lauric acid, directly increase blood LDL-cholesterol levels in a linear manner[13]. LDL-cholesterol is a direct contributor to the development of atherosclerosis. Although the counter argument has been that coconut oil increases the 'good' cholesterol, HDL-cholesterol, there is no scientific evidence to support a benefit for preventing CVD or improving outcomes[14]. Lauric acid is classed as a medium-chain fatty acid, yet it acts more like a long-chain fatty acid and most certainly does elevate LDL-cholesterol. The worry is that many processed vegan foods now contain quite a bit of coconut oil. These foods should be eaten rarely, as a treat, as their long-term effects on health are unlikely to be favourable. So, coconut oil is best reserved for external use on skin and hair.

10.3 If B12 is only found in animal foods, doesn't that mean we should eat animals?

Vitamin B12 is only found in animal food, or so we keep being told. This is only partly true. Certainly, the main source of vitamin B12 in omnivorous diets is meat, eggs and dairy. It turns out that B12 is not made by the animals themselves but by bacteria in soil and water and to some extent by bacteria in the gut. Traditionally, human and non-human animals got vitamin B12 from eating plants and water contaminated by B12-producing bacteria. Given our modern food hygiene standards and water sanitation, this is no longer a major source of vitamin B12.

Vitamin B12 in animal foods

Ruminant animals utilise the mineral cobalt to make vitamin B12 and cobalt is added to animal feed, since their industrially-produced diets are inadequate without it[15]. Poultry and pig feeds are usually supplemented with vitamin B12; in fact, the majority of the B12 supplements produced in the world are fed to livestock[16]. Therefore, the fact that humans also require a vitamin B12 supplement when following a 100% plant-based diet does not provide a good argument against this diet pattern.

Vitamin B12 in older adults

In the US, it is recommended that all adults over the age of 50 years, regardless of diet pattern, supplement with vitamin B12 as ageing seems to be the most important risk factor for vitamin B12 deficiency[17, 18]. There are a number of reasons for this, including reduced production of stomach acid required for absorption of vitamin B12 and frequent use of medications that interfere with absorption, such as acid blockers for indigestion and metformin for type 2 diabetes. We can tell you from our clinical experience that most people seen in haematology clinics with vitamin B12 deficiency are not following a vegan diet. In fact, The Framingham Offspring Study (FOS) that examined the B12 status of 2999 omnivores of ages ranging from 26 to 83 found that 39% of study participants had blood levels of vitamin B12 in the 'low normal' to deficient range[19].

Vitamin B12 in duckweed

We now know that duckweed (also called water lentils), the smallest plant on earth, not only contains all nine essential amino acids, fibre, iron, zinc and polyphenols, but is also a source of vitamin B12. Studies are beginning to be published evaluating the role of duckweed in the diet and, in particular, a high-protein strain called Mankai. A randomised controlled study (RCT) of Mankai in 36 men did show that Mankai could increase blood vitamin B12 levels[20]. However, studies to date have not confirmed if this B12 is active in the body and suitable for correcting B12 deficiency. So, it's not quite the time to ditch B12 supplements.

There have been some interesting studies using Mankai as part of the Mediterranean diet, along with green tea and walnuts – the so-called 'green-Mediterranean diet'. In randomised studies, this enhanced Mediterranean diet was shown to be better at improving cardiovascular risk factors, including reducing body weight, blood pressure, cholesterol and high sensitivity C-reactive protein (CRP)[21]. In addition, it was more effective at treating fatty liver disease[22]. It's worth noting that the green-Mediterranean diet also limits red and processed meat more than the standard Mediterranean diet, replacing this with plant foods. One does wonder therefore how much the Mankai was contributing to the observed benefits other than adding an expense. Four servings at the time of writing costs US$45.00. Nonetheless, it does show that duckweed may find its place in a plant-based diet with the potential to be a dietary non-animal source of vitamin B12 too.

Vitamin B12 recommendations for vegans

Vegans and those on a 100% plant-based diet require a regular and reliable source of vitamin B12. The easiest way to obtain it is by taking a supplement. There are different formulations and dosing schedules that can be used. The most common forms are cyanocobalamin (cyanCbl) and methylcobalamin (methylCbl). MethylCbl is the active form of the vitamin but it is still disassembled by the body after consumption and then reassembled prior to use. CyanCbl is a synthetic compound that is more shelf-stable but requires conversion to the active form prior to use in the body. There may be some very rare reasons why a cyanide-containing form of B12 is not desirable – for example, in severe renal failure.

Vitamin B12 binds to transcobalamin (holoTC) and is thereby available for use by cells. HoloTC is a much better predictor of B12 status than total B12 and blood levels become reduced prior to any clinical consequences of B12 deficiency[23].

Vitamin B12 absorption is an extremely complex process and it is known that the intake of supplements is optimal either in lower and more frequent doses (when absorption is mainly achieved with the help of intrinsic factor, produced in a healthy stomach), or in high doses once or twice a week (when absorption with intrinsic factor is saturated and therefore relies on passive diffusion).

A study including 42 vegans – 25 men and 17 women – with an average age of 34 years, investigated the effectiveness of two forms of vitamin B12 in maintaining holoTC within the normal range [24]. The participants fell into three groups based on the type of vitamin B12 supplementation: vegans who supplemented with cyanCbl (group 1, n=21), vegans who supplemented with methylCbl (group 2, n=14) and vegans who supplemented with products identified as 'natural' which they had read were and/or believed to be rich in B12 (algae, kombucha, borscht, yeast) (group 3, n=7). The impact of frequency of supplementation was also investigated. The results showed that holoTC values were significantly higher in the group that supplemented using cyanCbl. Frequency of consumption was also a factor in predicting holoTC levels, with those supplementing daily having a higher level compared with those supplementing once or twice per week. HoloTC levels were much lower in group 3 (natural forms). On the basis of these results, it appears that cyanoCbl taken daily is the best way to obtain vitamin B12 on a vegan diet.

The usual recommended dose is at least 25-50 micrograms per day as an oral tablet, with older adults requiring higher doses. Sublingual formulations and forms that dissolve in the mouth (tablet or spray) are also available and a dose of 50 micrograms of these per day is an adequate way for vegans to obtain vitamin B12[25].

10.4 Why do people say plant foods contain anti-nutrients?

The term 'anti-nutrients' is used to describe compounds in food that block the absorption of other nutrients. How much they actually affect absorption of nutrients can be difficult to study as this will vary between people and be influenced by how the food is prepared and cooked. The levels of these anti-nutrients can also vary within the same food, based on the climate and environment they were grown in and the health of the soil. Commonly cited anti-nutrients that cause concern include:

- **Glucosinolates**, found in cruciferous vegetables, can prevent iodine absorption and cause problems with thyroid function.
- **Lectins** found in most plant foods, but particularly in beans and whole grains, are discussed in section 8.2 and can inhibit the absorption of calcium, iron, phosphorus and zinc.
- **Oxalates**, found in certain leafy greens, such as spinach, Swiss chard and beet greens, can inhibit the absorption of calcium.
- **Phytates**, found in whole grains, legumes and nuts, can inhibit the absorption of iron, zinc, magnesium and calcium.
- **Tannins**, found in tea, coffee and cocoa, can inhibit the absorption of iron.

Based on this list it may seem we are suggesting the avoidance of all the healthiest foods on the planet. Far from it – 'anti-nutrient' is a misleading term and does not take into account the action of the whole food and that these so-called anti-nutrients have many protective functions. For example, phytates, or 'phytic acid', in beans and whole grains have antioxidant properties and are one of the reasons bean consumption is thought to be protective against cancer development and other chronic illness[26].

As with the message of this whole book, it is best to concentrate on eating an overall healthy diet with a wide variety of whole plant foods rather than getting bogged down with concerns over individual foods and nutrients.

In reality, micronutrient deficiencies are no more likely on a plant-based diet than they are on an omnivorous diet. In the EPIC-Oxford study, when comparing intakes of various nutrients between different dietary patterns, the only nutrient intakes that were lower than recommended in those who avoided all animal products were vitamin B12 and calcium[27]. In the Adventist Health Study 2, low intakes of vitamin B12 was the main concern in the vegan group[28]. In both cohorts, vegans had lower than recommended vitamin D intakes, but this is an issue for all dietary patterns, especially when exposure to sunshine is inadequate, such as in the winter months. Zinc intake is generally lower in people who avoid meat consumption but it does not appear that zinc levels in vegetarians are low enough to cause deficiency and there has been no suggestion of long-term harm[26, 27].

Iodine intake does need some planning on a 100% plant-based diet as discussed in section 3.2, but with adequate intake cruciferous vegetables pose no problem for thyroid health. To improve nutrient absorption from foods, such as whole grains and beans, and reduce the impact of so-called anti-nutrients, it is best to soak them overnight and then cook properly. Sprouting, fermentation and pickling can also reduce the levels of compounds such as phytates.

10.5 But vitamin A is only found in animal foods?

This is only partially correct. Pre-formed vitamin A is found only in animal-derived foods, but this does not pose a problem because precursor compounds to vitamin A are found in plant foods.

Vitamin A is an umbrella term for a large number of related compounds also known as retinoids (e.g. retinol, retinal and retinoic acid)[31]. They can be differentiated into two groups depending on whether the food source is an animal or a plant. Vitamin A derived from animal-based foods is retinol (also called 'pre-formed vitamin A'), which is a yellow, fat-soluble compound that is the precursor to the most active form of vitamin A, retinoic acid. The form of vitamin A found in fruit and vegetables is called 'provitamin A carotenoid', which includes beta-carotene, alpha-carotene and beta-cryptoxanthin, and can be converted into retinol in the body. Although some carotenoids are not precursors to vitamin A, including lutein, zeaxanthin and lycopene, they are still beneficial to health.

Beta-carotene is the most abundant provitamin A carotenoid in plant foods and is found in yellow, red and green (leafy) vegetables, such as spinach, carrots, sweet potatoes and red peppers, and in yellow fruit, such as mango, papaya and apricots. Various factors influence the absorption and conversion of dietary carotenoids into vitamin A, including genetic variations[32]. Consuming carotenoid-rich foods with a healthy source of fat increases absorption and conversion[33]. Including carotenoid-rich foods in the diet on a daily basis is usually sufficient to obtain enough vitamin A.

10.6 Don't I need choline from animal foods for brain health?

In the summer of 2019, a rather controversial opinion piece about the lower choline content of plant-based diets was published in the journal, the *British Medical Journal: Nutrition, Prevention and Health*[34]. The article suggested that there is a looming 'choline crisis', with implications for brain health. Foods with the highest levels of choline are meat, fish, eggs and dairy. The media latched onto the article and published rather misleading stories suggesting vegans were risking their brain health due to lack of choline in their diet. Of note, the author of the *BMJ* article, Emma Derbyshire, is a member of the Meat Advisory Panel, a conflict of interest, which was not disclosed in the original publication and led to several revisions of the article after many people complained. Luckily, the Physicians' Committee for Responsible Medicine (PCRM) and the UK Vegan Society put the record straight, publishing statements in response. There is no evidence that plant-based diets are deficient in choline or increase the risk of cognitive impairment. In fact the opposite may be true, with non-meat eaters having a lower risk of dementia[35].

No dietary targets for choline intake have been set in the UK. In the US, the recommended daily intake is 550 milligrams for men and 425 milligrams for women, although the intake is lower in most people[36]. The European Food Standards Agency has set 400 mg as an adequate intake for adults[37].

Studies have actually shown that choline from meat and eggs is converted to trimethylamine by gut bacteria and, once absorbed, the liver converts this to trimethylamine oxide (TMAO), which has been associated with an increased risk of cardiovascular disease (CVD), type 2 diabetes and renal failure[35, 36, 37, 38]. In fact, cardiovascular disease and its risk factors are strong predictors of the risk of dementia in later life[42]. We know that vegans and vegetarians have a significantly lower risk of CVD than meat eaters[43]. We also know that meat-based diets are associated with higher levels of TMAO[44].

A subsequent response to the above mentioned opinion piece examined the association of choline intake with cardio-metabolic and all-cause mortality in three prospective studies, including 49,858 black, 23,766 white and 134,001 Chinese participants[45]. During a median follow up of 11.7 years, 28,673 deaths were identified, including 11,141 cardio-metabolic deaths. The study found that high intakes of total choline and certain choline-containing compounds were associated with increased risk of cardio-metabolic mortality, especially from diabetes and ischaemic heart disease. Although the mechanism of this association was not possible to establish, the authors concluded that it might be beneficial to reduce choline intake by 'replacing major food sources of choline (i.e. red meat and eggs) with plant-based foods (e.g. vegetables, nuts, and legumes)'.

Choline may indeed be important for brain health, but there is no evidence to support the fact that choline in the diet needs to come from animal foods and there are many reasons why it is best obtained from plant sources. Choline is present in the cell membranes of all plants and animals. As with many nutrients, more is not always better. It is perfectly possible to obtain enough from whole plant sources, with soya, quinoa, Brussels sprouts and broccoli being some of the best sources. In fact, soya contains more choline than chicken or fish[36].

10.7 If I am 100% plant-based, do I need to take an omega-3 supplement?

There is no clear-cut answer to this question. The only exception is for pregnant and lactating women, who should indeed take a supplement. For the rest of us, the jury is still out. Many plant-based physicians have been recommending a DHA/EPA algae-derived supplement for all those following a 100% whole-food plant-based diet, especially in older adults, due to potential benefits for brain health. However, there has been no long-term study of vegans that has actually demonstrated an increased risk of mood disorders or dementia due to a lack of long chain omega-3 fatty acids. We also don't know whether supplementation could improve upon the already excellent cardiovascular outcomes in people following a plant-based diet as such a study has not been performed.

There has also never been a study examining the effect of omega-3 fatty acid supplementation in vegans. So, for now, we are going to have to make decisions based on individual circumstances. If you find it difficult to consume a regular source of short-chain omega-3 fats, such as walnuts or flaxseeds, then the safest option is probably to take an algae supplement.

10.8 I have heard that plant foods have lower levels of vitamins now than they used to, so shouldn't I take supplements?

Based on reading this and other chapters you will have learnt that if you are eating a varied whole-food plant-based diet, you will have equivalent if not better levels of most important nutrients. We would recommend vitamin D3 and B12 supplements, understanding this recommendation is not just limited to those eating predominantly plant-based diets. We suggest paying attention to calcium intake as discussed in section 3.1, omega-3 supplementation as discussed above in section 10.7, and iodine as discussed in section 3.2.

Chapter 11

Common health concerns about vegan and vegetarian diets

11.1 Wasn't there a study that showed vegetarians and vegans had an increased risk of stroke?

There are two types of stroke: haemorrhagic (a bleed on the brain) and ischaemic (interrupted blood flow to the brain). The vast majority are ischaemic (more than 85-90%) and share the same risk factors as ischaemic heart disease. Stroke represents a huge health burden globally. The Global Burden of Disease study reported that, from the age of 25 years onwards, one in four people will have a stroke[1]. The INTERSTROKE study, an international case-control study of almost 27,000 participants, found that about 90% of stroke risk is associated with 10 potentially modifiable risk factors — hypertension, smoking, diabetes, physical activity, diet, psychosocial factors, abdominal obesity, alcohol, cardiac causes (including atrial fibrillation, myocardial infarction) and dyslipidaemia[2].

The data supporting a whole food plant-based diet for prevention and treatment of stroke are not as strong as for ischaemic heart disease, partly because research into this topic has not been as extensive[3]. Nevertheless, some broad observations can be made. Those eating more fruit and vegetables and less meat have a lower incidence of ischaemic stroke. Diet patterns that emphasise whole plant foods and minimise animal-derived foods, such as the DASH (Dietary Approaches to Stop Hypertension) and Mediterranean diet patterns, have been associated with a lower risk of stroke[4, 5].

Concerns have been raised about the impact of plant-based diets on the risk of stroke based on a 2019 report from the EPIC-Oxford study[6]. The study analysed participants on a vegetarian and vegan diet together as the number of cases in the vegan group alone was too small for meaningful statistics. The data showed an increased risk of haemorrhagic stroke in the vegetarians – three extra cases per 1000 population over 10 years – compared with meat and fish eaters. There was no impact of diet on the risk of ischaemic stroke. It should be noted that the study showed reduced risk of ischaemic heart disease in the vegetarian/vegan group; this amounted to 10 fewer cases of ischaemic heart disease per 1000 population over 10 years. So, the stats still favoured a vegetarian over a meat-based diet.

What should we make of these data? This is one paper from one prospective cohort. These results need to be confirmed before conclusions can be drawn. A meta-analysis and systematic review of prospective cohort studies from 2019 did not show an impact for a vegetarian diet pattern on the risk of stroke – neither positive nor negative impact – when compared with non-vegetarian diet patterns[7]. The vegetarian/vegan participants in the EPIC-Oxford cohort had sub-optimal levels of vitamin B12, vitamin D and long-chain omega-3 fats, which could have contributed to this observed increased risk of haemorrhagic stroke. Another explanation may be the low LDL-cholesterol in vegetarians and vegans, as studies have shown an increased risk of haemorrhagic stroke with lower LDL-cholesterol levels[8].

In contrast, a study reported in 2020 from a Taiwanese prospective cohort, including >13,000 participants, showed a significant reduction in ischaemic *and* haemorrhagic stroke in vegetarians[9]. Vegetarians had an approximately 60% reduction in risk of both types of stroke. This was despite lower vitamin B12 levels and mainly due to lower rates of hypertension. It should be noted that this cohort differed from the EPIC-Oxford one in that the Taiwanese Buddhists didn't smoke or drink alcohol and ate more soya foods.

A more recent study from 2021 analysed diet data from more than 200,000 men and women in the Health Professionals Follow-up Study and the Nurses' Health Study using the Plant Based Diet Index[10]. These participants had been followed prospectively for more than 30 years. The results showed that those participants who were most adherent to a *healthy* plant-based diet had a 10% reduction in all forms of stroke and there was no signal for increased risk of haemorrhagic stroke.

We can therefore conclude with the following:

- The prevalence of stroke is increasing, with one in four people experiencing a stroke in their lifetime
- Ischaemic stroke is by far the commonest form of stroke and shares the same risk factors as ischaemic heart disease, which are all improved on a plant-based diet
- Eating more dietary fibre, especially from fruit and vegetables, can significantly reduce the risk of ischaemic stroke with additional benefits for prevention of high blood pressure, heart disease, cancer and type 2 diabetes
- Red and processed meat consumption has consistently been associated with an increased risk of ischaemic stroke[11]
- More data are needed to make a conclusion on the impact of vegetarian and vegan diets on stroke risk
- The benefits to heart health far outweigh any potential increase in haemorrhagic stroke risk with a vegetarian or vegan diet.

11.2 Will a plant-based diet affect my child's development?

A number of national and international healthcare organisations, including the Academy of Nutrition and Dietetics in the US[12], the British Dietetic Association[13], the Canadian Pediatric Society[14] and the Scientific Society for Vegetarian Nutrition in Italy[15], have stated that appropriately planned vegetarian, including vegan, diets are healthful and nutritionally adequate for all stages of life including infancy, childhood and adolescence. We also know that many of our chronic diseases start in childhood, including obesity, heart disease and type 2 diabetes, suggesting that the earlier we start with whole-food plant-based nutrition the better. For example, high LDL-cholesterol levels in adolescence have a strong association with atherosclerosis later in life[16]. In fact, atherosclerosis has been shown to start in the womb when mothers have a high cholesterol level during pregnancy[17]. The diagnosis of type 2 diabetes is being made at a younger age and the incidence is rising in children, a trend entirely driven by unhealthy diets and sedentary lifestyles[18].

Although the available scientific literature on raising plant-based children is not as extensive as that for adults, the data we have confirms that a plant-based diet can adequately support growth and development in children with definite advantages for cardio-metabolic health as shown by healthier body weight and lower cholesterol levels[19]. In addition, vegan children tend to consume more fibre, unsaturated fats, vitamin C, folate, carotenoids, magnesium and potassium, whilst consuming lower levels of sugar and saturated fat.

The VeChi diet study from Germany provides contemporary data on health outcomes of children raised on a vegetarian and vegan diet. The study assessed the energy and macronutrient intake and growth of 430 children aged 1-3 years following either an omnivorous, vegetarian or vegan diet[20]. The results showed no significant differences in calorie intake, height or weight between the different diet groups. Protein requirements were easily met. Fat and added sugar intake were higher in children following an omnivorous diet and fibre intake higher in children following a vegan diet. Omnivores were also more likely to be overweight. The VeChi Youth Study of 149 vegetarian, 115 vegan and 137 omnivore children aged between 6 and 18 years similarly showed no specific nutritional risks in vegans and vegetarians compared with omnivores, and most vegan children were appropriately supplementing with vitamin B12[21]. All diet groups, including vegans, exceeded protein requirements. As expected, vegan children consumed more fibre and unsaturated fats and less saturated fat. Interestingly, all diet groups had a similar percentage of participants with vitamin B2 (riboflavin) and D3 levels below the reference range.

Some but not all studies have shown that vegan children may be lighter and shorter than omnivores, but still within the normal reference range[22, 23, 24]. Studies in older children have shown similar findings and overall no concern regarding growth or development in vegetarian and vegan children[25, 26].

Concerns over the appropriateness of soya formulas for vegan babies (and those with cow's milk allergy) where breastfeeding has not been possible still linger in the medical literature. Both Canada and the United Kingdom remain cautious about using soya formulas prior to 6 months of age[27, 28, 29]. This concern seems to be unfounded based on decades of research. A review of 35 studies spanning 104 years (1909 to July 2013) found no adverse impact on children's growth or development with the use of soya formulas[30]. Concerns regarding accelerated puberty were also unfounded[31, 32].

Care needs to be taken to ensure children following a 100% plant-based diet are meeting micronutrients needs. Vitamin B12 needs to be supplemented. Calcium intakes are generally lower in vegan children, and attention needs to be paid to ensuring adequate intake with fortified foods and plant drinks being a useful addition to the diet. Concerns regarding iron and zinc intake do not appear to be a genuine issue based on the available data[19, 33, 34, 35]. Although ferritin – body iron stores – may be lower in vegan children, as they are in vegan adults, this does not appear to put children at higher risk of iron deficiency per se when compared with omnivores[36]. Plant-based diets of course have an abundance of other nutrients that are beneficial to children, including folate, vitamin E, vitamin C and fibre, and are naturally low in saturated fat and cholesterol, with studies showing that children avoiding meat consumption have a lower blood cholesterol level[37, 38].

11.3 There are many published cases of children dying because of a vegan diet. What do you say about this?

The media love to highlight scare stories about babies and children who have become unwell or even died because they were being raised on a vegan diet. There have even been arrests and charges brought against vegan parents. Even medical journals have a tendency to publish case reports of adverse health outcomes in vegan children. However, when you delve below the headlines and analyse the diet these children were eating, it is never a healthy, balanced plant-based diet and often nothing to do with being vegan. Most commonly it is due to parents feeding their child a very restrictive diet that does not meet their energy or nutritional requirements. For example, in 2019 the media reported that vegan parents in Florida had been charged with the murder of their 18-month-old son due to malnutrition. The child was mainly being fed raw fruit and vegetables[39]. This would not be considered an appropriately planned plant-based diet. A similar case in Australia was reported in 2019 when a 20-month-old daughter of vegan parents was found to be severely malnourished and suffering from rickets due to being 'fed a diet of oats, potatoes, rice, tofu, bread, peanut butter and rice milk, with small snacks of fruit and vegetables'[40]. Once again, this is not an appropriately planned diet and rice milk is not recommended for children. There are numerous similar reports, but you get the idea. Any poorly planned diet has adverse consequences for children, regardless of whether meat and dairy products are included.

Similarly, in the medical literature there are deaths reported in vegan children for a variety of reasons, but this is largely because the diet was poorly planned and executed. Reasons include raising children on a raw vegan diet[41, 42], insufficient vitamin D intake leading to rickets[43] and vitamin B12 deficiency[44]. However, raw vegan diets are not recommended for children due to concerns around micronutrient deficiencies and being too bulky to provide enough calories. Vitamin D deficiency is not specific to children on a vegan diet, and the NHS in the UK advises vitamin D supplementation for all breastfed babies and children aged 1-4 years regardless of diet pattern. The same recommendation exists in Canada. Of course, vitamin B12 does need to be provided as a supplement in the vegan diet but, with appropriate education, parents can easily incorporate this into their child's diet.

Unfortunately, some nation-based medical organisations have taken a view based on these isolated cases that vegan diets are not safe for children. In 2019, the Royal Academy of Medicine of Belgium published a report suggesting that vegan diets were 'unsuitable for unborn children, children, teenagers, and pregnant and lactating women' and parents raising vegan children should be prosecuted. The report was poorly referenced and contained factually inaccurate information, including myths about vegan diets that have long been discredited. Sadly, reports such as these will only lead to parents avoiding support from healthcare professionals because they are less likely to tell their doctor that they are raising vegan children and may even lead to missed medical appointments in fear of facing inappropriate criminal charges.

11.4 What about plant-based diets for adolescents and teenagers?

We already know that healthy plant-based diets can support all stages of life, but what does the science tell us about the health and diet quality of adolescents and teenagers? Again, the data in this area are not extensive. The VeChi youth study (discussed in section 11.2) included children up to 18 years of age and confirmed the adequacy of a well-planned vegan diet[21]. The Teen Food and Development Study was conducted among adolescents to examine associations between dietary intake and health outcomes[45]. It included 601 adolescents (262 males and 339 females) aged 12–18 years in a predominantly Adventist population in the US. The study examined the diet of vegetarian and non-vegetarian participants. Overall, the results showed that diet quality was better in the vegetarians, with greater intakes of foods considered to be beneficial to health and an overall better nutrient intake profile, including lower, yet adequate calorie intakes, lower consumption of saturated fat, a more favorable omega-6 to omega-3 ratio, and higher intakes of dietary fibre, potassium and magnesium, folate, iron and calcium. However, there was a concern that vegetarian diets were still higher in salt than the recommended intake, a reflection of processed and pre-packaged food consumption.

The same study has also shown that consumption of animal protein in this age group is associated with higher body weight and greater risk of obesity, including the unhealthiest type of obesity with fat deposition around the abdomen[46]. An earlier study from the US including 4756 adolescents, with more than half of participants being from non-white backgrounds, demonstrated that the 262 vegetarian participants were consuming a diet of higher quality with a better nutritional profile than the non-vegetarian participants[47]. Most of these studies include very few children consuming a vegan diet, but there does not seem to be a particular concern in relation to removing dairy and eggs from the diet assuming due care is taken to ensure adequate intakes of vitamin B12, vitamin D, calcium and iodine[48, 49].

There are several further benefits of a plant-based diet for children. Avoidance of dairy significantly reduces the incidence of acne as dairy increases blood insulin and insulin-like growth factor levels (IGF-1), which are implicated in the development of acne[50]. Including regular consumption of soya foods, such as tofu, in childhood and adolescence has been associated with a lower risk of breast cancer in women later in life[51]. The lower cholesterol and saturated fat intake promotes better future cardiovascular health[16]. The ability to maintain a healthier weight with a plant-based diet reduces the risk of developing type 2 diabetes[52].

Diet and puberty

There is some evidence to support a dietary influence over the timing of puberty, although the data are by no means consistent. In general, studies show a later onset of menarche (first period) in girls who avoid meat consumption and an earlier onset in those who are overweight and consuming the most red meat or poultry[53, 54, 55, 56, 57]. There are some reported benefits to a later onset of menarche, including a lower risk of breast cancer[58], cardiovascular disease (CVD)[59], type 2 diabetes[60] and migraines[61]. However, late menarche may be a risk factor for osteoporosis given the shorter lifetime exposure to oestrogens[62].

There do not appear to be major differences in puberty onset for boys based on the consumption or avoidance of animal foods. However, in general, a better diet quality, including choosing vegetable protein over animal sources, is associated with later onset of puberty for boys and girls[63, 64].

11.5 Does being vegan or vegetarian predispose you to eating disorders?

It is a commonly expressed belief that being vegan or vegetarian predisposes you to eating disorders, but not one we agree with. This is not to say that vegetarians or vegans cannot suffer from eating disorders; they can, of course. Eating disorders are a serious mental illness with complex causes and manifestations. They are not a lifestyle choice. The suggestion that vegetarianism predisposes to eating disorders came from studies that described a high prevalence of disordered eating behaviours in vegetarians[65, 66]. A systematic review of 20 studies concluded that there was a correlation between vegetarianism and the presence of eating disorders[67]. However, the authors stated that most studies were of a cross-sectional design, and so could not clarify a causal relationship between vegetarianism and disordered eating. Other limitations included a lack of differentiation of eating disorder diagnoses and variability in the definitions of vegetarianism. Reverse causation has to be considered – that is, did the experience of an eating disorder come first or did it manifest following a decision to follow a vegetarian diet pattern?

Several studies looking at this question have shown that in the majority of the population studied, identifying as vegetarian came *after* the diagnosis of the eating disorder[68, 69]. The more pertinent question is not whether being vegetarian predisposes to an eating disorder but whether there is a higher prevalence of identifying as vegetarian in people who suffer from eating disorders compared with those who do not, and this does seem to be the case[68].

There are a variety of reasons behind someone's choice to become vegetarian, weight loss being one of them, sometimes termed 'pseudo-vegetarianism'[69]. Identifying as vegetarian may be a socially acceptable way to avoid certain foods and restrict calories.

What about vegans? One study looked at eating and health-related attitudes and behaviours in 345 vegans compared with 220 omnivores[70]. Vegans scored significantly better than omnivores on the Eating Disorder Examination Questionnaire, which is a measure of pathological eating behaviour. The authors concluded that, in general, vegans did not differ from omnivores in their eating attitudes and behaviours, but where they did differ, they showed healthier attitudes and behaviours towards food, including in cooking more at home, consuming more fruit, vegetables, nuts, beans and grains, and consuming fewer caffeinated soft drinks.

The Academy of Dietetics and Nutrition sums this issue up nicely in their 2016 position paper on vegetarian diets: 'Eating disorders have a complex aetiology and prior use of a vegetarian or vegan diet does not appear to increase the risk of an eating disorder, though some with pre-existing disordered eating may choose these diets to aid their limitation of food intake.'[71]

11.6 Can I have a healthy pregnancy on a plant-based diet?

The unique nutritional requirements during pregnancy and lactation often lead to questions about the safety of vegan and vegetarian diets in these situations. However, the scientific consensus is that a healthy plant-based diet can adequately support these life stages and may even have some advantages for mother and baby. Again, it comes down to having the right knowledge and support, and to planning ahead, as with any pregnancy. Available evidence suggests that well-planned vegan and vegetarian diets, with attention to the specific nutrients, are safe in pregnancy, lactation and childhood[71, 72].

For mothers who are consuming a 100% plant-based or vegan diet, vitamin B12 supplementation is essential. Vitamin D supplementation is often required, especially when sun exposure is limited. Iodine is usually also required in supplement form, depending on the iodine content of the mother's diet. In addition, supplementation with long-chain omega-3 fatty acids (EPA/ DHA) are recommended to help prevent preterm labour and for the baby's neurological development.

Protein requirements increase in the third trimester, so emphasising protein-rich plant foods at every meal, such as beans and legumes, soya milk, tofu, tempeh, nuts and seeds, is helpful. It is also important to obtain enough calcium as this may help prevent pre-eclampsia (high blood pressure in pregnancy). Foods high in calcium, such as calcium-set tofu, fortified plant milks and yoghurts, green vegetables (collard greens, kale, spring greens, bok choy, broccoli, rocket), chia and sesame seeds, almonds and beans, are useful to include on a daily basis.

Vegan and vegetarian diets may also reduce the risk of certain pregnancy-related conditions, such as excessive weight gain, pre-eclampsia and gestational diabetes[72]. Optimising a mother's cardiovascular health during pregnancy, with healthier weight and optimal blood glucose and cholesterol levels, can reduce the future risk of CVD in offspring[73]. We know a plant-based diet is the most effective dietary approach to achieve this.

11.7 Elders need animal protein to prevent muscle and bone loss, don't they?

There are some specific nutritional issues to consider with regard to plant-based diets for older adults. In general, energy/calorie requirements decrease with age as a result of a reduced basal metabolic rate but the requirements for other essential nutrients may actually increase. It is generally accepted that elders, or those over the age of 65 years, may need to eat more protein to prevent age-related muscle loss (sarcopenia), osteoporosis and general frailty. Overweight is also an increasing issue, and this can co-exist with low muscle mass[74].

Although this remains a topic of debate, the European clinical guidelines for older adults recommend a protein intake of at least 1 gram of protein per kilogram of body weight per day and 1–1.2 grams per day is thought to be good to aim for[75]. This higher intake of protein has usually been assumed to be best obtained from meat. However, this concept is changing given the enormous benefits to health for adults less than 65 years of obtaining protein predominantly from plant sources[76]. This is likely in part to be due to the fact that plant foods in general reduce oxidative stress and inflammation, two key processes involved in the ageing process, sometimes referred to as 'inflammaging'[77]. In addition, removing red and processed meat from the diet appears particularly favourable for all age groups, including elders, as red meat consumption has been associated with an increased risk of dying early from CVD and cancer[78].

The increased risk of sarcopenia and frailty with ageing is in turn a risk factor for falls and fractures, disability, reduced quality of life and reduced life expectancy. We now spend on average at least 10 years with ill health before we die[79]. The science supports healthy lifestyle behaviours for the prevention of chronic illness with ageing. When it comes to diet, studies have shown that dietary factors that prevent sarcopenia and frailty and reduce the chances of premature death include an overall healthy diet pattern that is predominantly plant-based[80], emphasises plant protein over animal protein[81] and includes plenty of whole grains[82] and fruit and vegetables[83]. That's essentially a whole food plant-based diet.

Various other nutrients are important for healthy ageing and requirements for some may increase as we get older, including calcium, vitamin B12, vitamin D and long-chain omega-3 fats[74]. There is continued belief amongst health professionals that dairy is required to meet calcium requirements as we age, mainly because of the need for adequate calcium intake for bone health. However, studies have not confirmed that dairy consumption leads to better bone health. In fact, when you delve into the science, some studies have actually shown a higher incidence of hip fracture, a good marker of osteoporosis, in countries that consume the highest amount of dairy, like Sweden[84]. Although this does not prove cause and effect, it also does not prove the essentiality of dairy for bone health. Overall, the science does not support high intakes of dairy for prevention of osteoporosis.

Foods most associated with better bone health are fruit and vegetables, which as a society we are just not consuming enough of, and of course an adequate intake of calcium and vitamin D[85]. Avoidance of added salt, tobacco smoking, caffeine and alcohol is beneficial, and the most effective way to preserve our bone health as we age is weight-bearing and muscle strengthening exercises.

11.8 What about prevention of dementia? Don't we need nutrients from animal foods?

The rising burden of dementia is a global problem and its impact in the coming decades is going to be felt more in low- and middle-income countries. Worldwide around 50 million people live with dementia, and this number is projected to increase to 152 million by 2050. The Lancet Commission on Dementia has done an excellent job at highlighting the impact of socioeconomic and lifestyle factors that contribute to the development of dementia. The first report was published in 2017 and then updated in 2020[86, 87]. The commission has identified 12 potentially modifiable factors that are thought to be important in preventing or delaying the onset of dementia in up to 40% of cases. These risk factors are: type 2 diabetes, obesity, hypertension, smoking, lack of physical activity, depression, hearing impairment, low educational attainment, social isolation, excessive alcohol consumption, air pollution and traumatic brain injury. It should be noted that the studies informing these recommendations were mostly performed in high-income countries, whereas the burden of dementia is greater in low- and middle-income countries and therefore the potential for prevention may be even greater.

Other contributing factors discussed in the report include good quality sleep and diet. Regarding diet, the focus of researchers has turned more to diet patterns rather than individual nutrients. High intake of whole plant foods is what the paper recommends. Data supporting the Mediterranean diet pattern is strongest because of the high consumption of fruit, vegetables, cereals, nuts, legumes and olive oil, with low intake of saturated fats and meat. This diet pattern is also recommended by the World Health Organization (WHO) for prevention of dementia[88].

There is no strong evidence for the use of supplements, but vitamin and other micronutrient consumption should be optimised through the diet. There are some individual nutrients and particular foods that are associated with a lower risk of the commonest type of dementia, Alzheimer's[89]. Vitamin E from food (nuts, oils, seeds, leafy green vegetables and whole grains) is consistently protective. If the diet is not optimal in vitamin E, then a supplement may be protective but there is no added benefit of supplements if vitamin E from the diet is optimal. Folate (vitamin B9, in vegetables and whole grains) and vitamin B12 are consistently protective. Vegetables (particularly green leafy) appear to be more important than fruit in protecting against Alzheimer dementia, with the exception of berry consumption, which appears highly protective against cognitive decline.

A recent study highlighted the importance of eating plenty of fruit and vegetables early in life to prevent later cognitive impairment[90]. This study recruited more than 3000 participants in the US aged 18 to 30 years in the 1980s and followed them for 25 years, regularly documenting their dietary intake. It found that those consuming the most fruit and vegetables in younger life had the best cognitive function later in life. In this study, vegetable consumption had a greater effect than fruit consumption, with particular nutrients such as lycopene from tomatoes / red vegetables and beta-carotene from yellow / orange vegetables having the best effect. Neither potato nor fruit juice consumption showed a benefit. Overall, it seemed that it was the fibre intake that was responsible for much of this beneficial effect on brain health.

Fibre intake is correlated with lower risk of many chronic diseases that increase the risk of dementia, such as CVD, type 2 diabetes and hyperlipidaemia. Fibre intake benefits gut bacteria, which then make short-chain fatty acids needed for brain hormone production and which reduce inflammation, key to preventing dementia[91].

Consumption of flavonoids from fruit and vegetables may be of particular benefit[92]. Flavonoids are a class of polyphenols representing more than 5000 bioactive compounds that are found in a variety of fruit and vegetables. Two papers reporting results from large prospective cohort studies from the US demonstrated that higher consumption of flavonoids may significantly reduce the risk of Alzheimer dementia and other dementias[93, 94]. Similarly, higher consumption of carotenoids, the naturally occurring pigments found in red, yellow, orange and dark green fruit and vegetables, has also been associated with a lower risk of Alzheimer dementia[95].

Overall, it can be said that it is mainly the plant foods in the diet that prevent dementia and the earlier in life you start a healthy diet the better it is for brain health. In fact, meat consumption in general is likely to be detrimental to brain health, mainly due to the saturated fat content and increased risk of chronic illnesses such as CVD and type 2 diabetes that increase the risk of dementia[89, 96]. The only exception to this is with the consumption of fish and the reported benefits of long-chain omega-3 fatty acids. DHA (a long-chain omega-3 fatty acid) is very important for the developing brain and has also been shown to be important in protecting the ageing brain.

The brain is composed of around 50-60% fat and has a particularly high content of DHA. Higher levels of DHA in the brain may be associated with better brain health[97]. Several studies have shown that the regular consumption of fish reduced the risk of dementia[98, 99]. However, whether fish consumption reflects a healthier diet in general, likely to be lower in harmful foods such as red and processed meat, or whether fish itself has nutrients, including long-chain omega-3 fatty acids, that are beneficial for brain health, is not clear. There are also concerns about exposure to heavy metal contaminants in fish (including mercury) and whether in the longer term we will begin to see an adverse impact on brain function. Supplementation with fish oils, high in omega-3 fatty acids, have not consistently been shown to prevent dementia[100]. Whether those who do not consume any seafood should supplement with an algae-derived DHA/EPA supplement is still in question but given the lack of harm, some plant-based healthcare professionals do advise older adults to take an algae-based supplement.

11.9 What about mental health? Haven't studies on people following vegan and vegetarian diets shown that they are more depressed?

A systematic review from 2021 concluded that people who avoid eating meat have a higher prevalence of depression, anxiety and/or self-harm behaviours[101]. This sounds rather alarming and of course made media headlines, but what should you know about the study before drawing any conclusions?

This study was funded in part via an unrestricted research grant from the Beef Checkoff, through the National Cattlemen's Beef Association. We know that studies sponsored by industry are more likely to find results in favour of their products, drugs or devices[102]. Food-industry-sponsored studies are no different.

Sixteen of the 18 studies included in the review are of cross-sectional design[103]. This is a weak study design as it examines a group of individuals at only one point in time. It cannot take into account what came first – the mental health disorder or removing meat from the diet. The review clearly states that for most studies they did not know which came first. Certainly, in one study, meat was excluded from the diet on average five years *after* the diagnosis of a mental health disorder. The authors clearly state that: 'There was no evidence to support a causal relation between the consumption or avoidance of meat and any psychological outcomes' for the reasons stated above.

Eleven of the 18 studies included showed a negative impact of meat abstinence on psychological well-being, four studies showed no impact and three showed a favourable impact. So, by no means did all studies included reach the same conclusion as the review article. The one randomised controlled trial (RCT – a more rigorous study design) of diet and mental health that was included actually showed *benefit* for a vegetarian diet pattern.

The quality of the diet in those who avoided meat consumption was not included. Vegetarians and vegans can live off ultra-processed foods, which we know can adversely affect mental health[104]. This cannot be extrapolated to conclude that a *healthy* vegetarian or vegan diet causes mental health disorders.

We have plenty of more robust data from prospective cohort studies demonstrating that diet patterns that increase the consumption of whole plant foods, especially fruit and vegetables, whilst minimising animal-derived foods, are associated with better mental health and well-being[105]. We have data from two randomised studies, the SMILES and the HELFIMED trials, that demonstrate the benefits of a Mediterranean diet pattern, which emphasises whole plant foods whilst minimising red and processed meat, for those with an established diagnosis of depression[106, 107]. We even have a randomised study examining the impact of a low-fat vegan diet in a multi-centre workplace intervention conducted by the PCRM (Physicians' Committee for Responsible Medicine) for the company GEICO in the US[108]. It is not clear why this study was not included in the systematic review. Altogether, 292 participants across 10 corporate sites, who were overweight and/or had a history of type 2 diabetes, were randomly allocated to follow a low-fat vegan diet composed of fruit, vegetables, whole grains and legumes, or to continue their usual diet for 18 weeks. The intervention group also had weekly support meetings. The results showed a significant improvement in mental health well-being and work productivity and reductions in depression and anxiety scores in those on the vegan diet. Because the study aimed to measure the effects of the vegan diet and a nutrition program in the workplace, the control group did not receive the weekly support meetings, which could have contributed to the beneficial findings in addition to the diet.

Overall, there are limited data on the long-term impact of vegan and vegetarian diets on mental health. However, given the importance of a healthy gut microbiome and the impact of chronic inflammation on mental health and well-being, it can be hypothesised that plant-based diets, which improve gut health and lower inflammation, may be beneficial[109, 110]. We accept that the role of fish in the diet for its impact on mental health remains a matter for debate[111]. For us, the level of heavy metal, plastic and toxin contamination of fish is reason enough to avoid fish and obtain long-chain omega-3 fatty acids directly from marine algae.

All in all, these misleading headlines were generated from a poorly conducted review, funded by the beef industry with an over-interpretation of the results in favour of the sponsors.

11.10 Can a plant-based diet reverse heart disease?

There is an ongoing debate in the plant-based community as to whether a plant-based diet can actually lead to regression of established atherosclerotic plaques in the arteries[112]. There is a definition in the cardiology community for clinically relevant plaque reversal, which has been used to test the efficacy of medications such as statins[113]. However, studies by Dr Esselstyn and Dr Ornish that are most widely cited as evidence for a plant-based diet to reverse coronary artery disease do not meet these strict newer criteria[114, 115].

What is clear is that for patients with established coronary artery disease, a plant-based diet can improve symptoms such as angina, significantly reduce the risk of further cardiovascular events and reduce the risk of dying from CVD. For us this is enough on its own to consider a plant-based diet as the optimal diet for those with heart disease. However, when you have established heart disease and have had a cardiovascular event, such as a heart attack or stroke, the benefits of a plant-based diet do not necessarily allow for the discontinuation of standard medical therapy such as statins or aspirin. Many patients are looking to come off medications such as statins, but statins have more than just a cholesterol-lowering effect. They also lead to plaque stabilisation and have anti-inflammatory properties. Nonetheless, being able to improve patient outcomes is the key to any intervention and a plant-based diet has been shown to do this. As doctors we like to use all the available tools to improve the health of our patients and it's clear that a plant-based diet, which can be 100% plant-based, should be included as part of the recovery from heart disease and for maintaining a good quality of life.

11.11 Why are there always stories about celebrities ditching their vegan diet because it made them feel ill?

The media love to jump on stories of vegans who have stopped being vegan, for clickbait and increased readership, propagating the myth that somehow a vegan diet is not healthy for humans.

Celebrities do indeed have a significant influence on popular culture, but these celebrities are not healthcare professionals, and one person's story does not change the huge body of evidence in favour of the health-promoting benefits of plant-based nutrition. There may be any number of reasons why someone, celebrity or not, may not feel in optimal health whilst on a vegan diet. A diet that omits animal products is not necessarily health promoting, and new vegans may substitute animal products with processed foods, and may not be getting enough whole plant foods, or perhaps not getting enough calories given the lower calorie density of plant foods.

Celebrities can also face the same significant social challenges from family and friends as the rest of us when becoming plant-based which can derail one's best intentions, and if one is not educated in the common misconceptions of plant-based nutrition it would be easy to listen to the unfounded concerns of others. We have certainly had to unlearn a lot of nutrition myths in our journey.

It is worth noting, as we have already discussed, that potential nutrient deficiencies in those on a plant-based diet are easy to correct – for example, in vitamins D and B12 – with supplementation.

11.12 How do we know vegan or vegetarian diets are healthy in the longer term?

We now have quite long follow-up data from several studies investigating the health impact of a plant-based diet. As explained in Chapter 1, we have studies such as the EPIC-Oxford study and the Adventist Health Studies that have investigated specifically the health of vegans and vegetarians. We also have results from large prospective cohort studies such as the Nurses' Health Study and the Health Professionals Follow-up Study from the US, and more recently the NutriNet Santé cohort from France that has analysed diet data using the Plant-Based Dietary Index to investigate the impact of plant-based diets on long-term health.

There are some general themes that have emerged. Those following a healthy plant-based diet, including vegetarian and vegan diets, have a significantly reduced risk of hypertension (up to 60% reduced risk compared with omnivores), high cholesterol (vegans are the only diet group that consistently maintains a healthy cholesterol level), heart disease (25% reduced risk) and type 2 diabetes (50% reduced risk)[116]. For cancer, when you combine the results from various studies on vegan and vegetarian health, vegans have overall a 15% reduction in risk of cancer; however, studies differ with regard to the risk based on specific cancer sites[117]. In the NutriNet Santé French Cohort, cancer risk was also reduced by 15% for those following the most healthy plant-based diet[118]. A healthy plant-based diet is associated with a 14% reduction in the risk of developing kidney failure[119] and a 10% reduction in the risk of stroke.

The million-dollar question is whether vegans and vegetarians live longer. The Adventist Health Study has shown an advantage for those avoiding meat consumption whereas the EPIC-Oxford has not. In part, this may be because the Adventist Health Study included generally health-conscious participants and thus even the meat eaters were healthier than the general UK population of EPIC-Oxford[116, 120]. When analysing dietary data using the Plant-Based Dietary Index, studies have shown a 5-10% reduction in the risk of death, meaning that those following a healthy plant-based diet may live longer than those consuming an animal-based diet[121, 122]. That's not bad in our view! The main point is that, regardless of whether a diet makes you live longer, we know that a plant-based diet will mean you have the best chance of living a healthy life, free of chronic illness.

11.13 But there isn't one diet that fits all because we all have differences in our genes?

It seems that the latest 'rabbit hole' that the nutrition community are going down is that of 'Precision Nutrition'. This is the concept that diet needs to be personalised and one diet pattern does not fit all. Our view is that this is taking the conversation away from what we already know about nutrition and health – that is, a diet centred on fruit, vegetables, whole grains, nuts and seeds is associated with the best health outcomes.

It has become 'fashionable' to measure individual glucose and insulin responses to common foods or analyse the gut microbiome and then come up with a specific diet for a particular individual. This concept has, however, been put to the test and for now is not supported by the weight of evidence. For example, a well-designed study called the DIETFITS (Diet Intervention Examining the Factors Interacting with Treatment Success) study investigated the impact of a healthy low-carb diet versus a healthy low-fat diet on weight loss and correlated the results with certain genetic markers that were supposed to predict for responses to fat and carbohydrate intake. Results were also correlated with the participants' insulin responses to a glucose load[123]. After 12 months, there was no significant difference in weight change between a healthy low-fat diet versus a healthy low-carbohydrate diet in the 609 participants. Both groups had been instructed to eat as many vegetables as possible, limit processed foods and added sugar, and eat home-cooked food. Neither the different genetic markers nor the insulin responses were able to predict for weight loss or were associated with the effectiveness of either diet pattern. The results instead emphasised the importance of food quality and a sustainable approach rather than a personalised diet.

Another example of a study attempting to examine personalised responses to foods is the PREDICT 1 (Personalised

REsponses to Dietary Composition Trial 1) trial, an international collaboration to study associations between diet, the microbiome and biomarkers of cardio-metabolic health[124]. The researchers collected microbiome sequence data, detailed long-term dietary information and the results of hundreds of cardio-metabolic blood markers from just over 1100 participants in the UK and US. The study examined markers of health such as BMI, weight, waist/hip ratio, blood pressure, visceral fat, antibiotic use, fasting and post-prandial lipid and glucose profiles, fatty acid metabolism and markers of inflammation. The results showed that the composition and diversity of the gut microbiome were strongly associated with specific foods and dietary patterns, which in turn were associated with blood and biometric measures of health.

In the study, the health of the microbiome and biomarkers had a greater association with dietary factors than with genetic factors, as evidenced by the inclusion of 480 monozygotic and dizygotic twins in the study population. The results showed that the health of the gut microbiome was strongly associated with the consumption of healthy plant foods with diversity and quality of the diet being the most important factors.

The bacterial composition associated with a healthy plant-predominant diet was linked with beneficial impacts on markers of cardio-metabolic health and inflammation that can predict for a lower risk of developing conditions such as obesity, type 2 diabetes and CVD. The converse was also true in that processed foods, refined carbohydrates and sugar, meat, animal fat and high-fat dairy foods were associated with a less healthy gut microbiome composition, which was associated with blood markers that predict for an increased risk of chronic disease.

This brings us back to the original point, that the vast majority of the world's population can thrive on a predominantly or entirely whole food plant-based diet and that this drastically reduces their future risk of chronic illness.

Chapter 12

Additional benefits of a plant-based diet

12.1 Prevention and treatment of fatty liver disease

Non-alcoholic fatty liver disease (NAFLD) is the accumulation of fat in the liver. When progressive, it can lead to liver fibrosis and cirrhosis. The incidence of NAFLD is rising, with up to 20% of Western populations having some evidence of NAFLD[1]. The key drivers are obesity, dyslipidaemia, insulin resistance and metabolic syndrome. These factors are intimately related to diet and lifestyle. The specific components of diet that are associated with an increased risk of NAFLD include saturated fat, red and processed meat, refined carbohydrates and fructose (from sugar and high-fructose corn syrup). Remarkably, NAFLD was not even recognised as a clinical entity prior to 1980, yet it is now one of the top reasons for performing a liver transplant. In the same period, meat and processed food consumption has increased as have obesity, diabetes and metabolic syndrome; NAFLD is considered to be the liver component of metabolic syndrome.

Healthy diet patterns, such as the Mediterranean diet, are associated with a lower risk of NAFLD[2]. A healthy plant-based diet when assessed using the plant-based diet index was assoc-iated with a 21% reduction in risk of NAFLD when compared with an omnivorous diet, but an unhealthy plant-based diet (made up of processed foods and refined carbohydrates) did not protect against NAFLD and in fact increased the risk[3].

The impact of vegetarian diets on the incidence of NAFLD was examined in the Tzu Chi Health Study from Taiwan[4]. This study included 2127 non-vegetarians and 1273 vegetarians who did not smoke or habitually drink alcohol and did not have hepatitis B or hepatitis C infection. Vegetarians had a 21% reduced risk of NAFLD. Replacing a serving of soya with a serving of meat or fish was associated with 12–13% increased risk, whereas replacing a serving of whole grains with a serving of refined grains, fruit and/or fruit juice was associated with 3–12% increased risk of NAFLD.

The impact of a vegan diet has been investigated in a small study that included 29 patients with NAFLD[5]. They adopted a vegan diet for six months, although four patients subsequently dropped out leaving 26 patients for evaluation. The results showed a significant reduction in weight (median 5 kilograms) and BMI (median 1.66 BMI points) and normalisation of liver function in 20 of 26 patients (76%). Four patients were also able to reduce medication dosage for their underlying cardio-metabolic diseases.

A larger study from researchers at the PCRM (Physicians' Committee for Responsible Medicine) randomly allocated 244 overweight or obese adults to a low-fat vegan diet or no dietary change for 16 weeks[6]. The results showed that the vegan group lowered their body weight by 6.4 kilograms (about 14 pounds/1 stone) and the fat inside the liver and muscle cells by 34% and 10%, respectively. They also increased their after-meal energy expenditure by 18.7%. There were no significant changes in the measured parameters in the control group. The decrease in liver and muscle fat correlated with improvements in insulin resistance.

Overall, a diet composed of healthy plant foods, whilst minimising animal foods and processed foods, is the best way to maintain liver health.

12.2 Prevention of kidney stones

About 10% of people develop kidney stones in their lifetime, most of whom are consuming an omnivorous diet. The most common composition of renal stones is calcium oxalate. In the EPIC-Oxford study, non-meat eaters had a significantly *reduced* risk of developing kidney stones – down 30-50% compared with meat-eaters[7]. Interestingly, higher zinc intake (associated with eating meat), was associated with a higher risk of kidney stones, whereas fruit and fibre intake was protective.

Although we don't have specific data on 100% plant-based or vegan diets and kidney stones, there remains a concern about the potentially high intake of oxalates from plant foods such as spinach, Swiss chard, nuts and beets. However, the relationship between intake and risk of stones is not straightforward. Other factors can increase the risk too, such as too much protein, not enough calcium, vitamin C supplements, too much salt and sugar, and dehydration. Certain underlying medical conditions can result in too much oxalate being absorbed from the gut.

You can of course optimise your plant-based diet to have a lower oxalate content by limiting some of the high-oxalate foods and making sure other aspects of your diet are optimised, including sufficient calcium, not too much salt and sugar and plenty of water for hydration[8].

12.3 Prevention of urinary tract infections

Urinary tract infections (UTIs) are one of the most common causes of infection in the general population, with the bacteria *Escherichia coli (E. coli)* often being the culprit. Infection can occur because *E. coli* from the intestine finds its way into the urinary tract. However, UTIs can also be caused by *E. coli* strains commonly found in farm animals, such as chickens and pigs, so eating contaminated sources of meat can lead to infection.

Given the link between *E. coli* and UTIs, it might seem obvious that those on a plant-based diet who avoid meat have a lower risk of infection. Analysis from the Tzu Chi Vegetarian Study of Taiwanese Buddhists showed that vegetarians had a 16% lower risk of UTIs compared with non-vegetarians[9]. This confirms previous data suggesting that meat-borne bacteria are a major contributor to the risk of UTIs. Increasingly these food-borne bacteria are also displaying antibiotic resistance[10].

12.4 Reduction of arthritic pain

Osteoarthritis, the painful breakdown of cartilage in the joints, appears to be an inevitable consequence of ageing. It is not reversible, but is manageable, usually with pain medication and sometimes surgery. One small, randomised study in patients with osteoarthritis put a whole-food plant-based diet to the test for six weeks[11]. Patients on a plant-based diet reported significant improvement in pain and functioning. The main reason is likely to be the anti-inflammatory properties of the micronutrients present in plant foods, as inflammation is the main cause of pain in arthritis[12]. Meat-based diets have the opposite effect and, in general, increase the level of inflammation in the body.

Does that include gout?

Another type of painful arthritis is gout, caused by elevated levels of uric acid which can form crystals and deposit in the joints. The main source of uric acid is from the breakdown of purines, compounds found at higher levels in meat and seafood compared with plant sources of food. In addition, the breakdown of fructose (from sugar-sweetened beverages and other processed foods, but not whole fruit) increases uric acid levels and hence the risk of gout.

Analysis of the risk of gout in almost 5000 participants in

the Tzu Chi Health Study and Tzu Chi Vegetarian Study found that vegetarians had a 40-60% significantly reduced risk of developing gout[13]. The beneficial effect of avoiding meat and fish consumption appeared to be at least in part independent of uric acid levels, suggesting that other aspects of a vegetarian diet, such as lower levels of inflammation, may also be important. Soya is often considered a high source of purine, but interestingly, soya consumption in this study was associated with a lower risk of gout, possibly due to the differences in the type of purines compared with meat and the ability of soya to reduce inflammation.

12.5 Reduction of period pain in women

So, if a plant-based diet can improve arthritis pain, could it also perhaps improve other types of pain? A crossover trial of 33 women put this to the test for menstrual pain and symptoms[14]. Women swapped to a low-fat vegan diet for two menstrual cycles, and then back to their usual omnivorous diet for their next two. Pain duration, intensity and premenstrual symptoms were recorded and levels of a protein that affects oestrogen levels were measured. On the low-fat vegan diet, women reported less pain duration and intensity and shorter duration of premenstrual symptoms and their blood tests showed a lower level of oestrogen.

People are often surprised to hear that diet can impact hormone levels in the body. This study shows exactly that, and how lower oestrogen levels can benefit women's health in several ways.

12.6 Alleviating menopausal symptoms

Peri- and post-menopausal symptoms can be a real challenge for women, adversely affecting their quality of life. Hot flashes are a particular problem. Many studies have suggested that diet and lifestyle habits are important in managing symptoms during this phase of life, with the potential to reduce or eliminate symptoms altogether. For the first time, we have a randomised study that tested the impact of a low-fat, healthy vegan diet based on fruits, vegetables, whole grains, and legumes and which minimised added oils and fatty foods (e.g. nuts, nut butters, avocado) with the addition of one portion (86 grams or half a cup) of cooked whole soyabeans per day[15]. Thirty-eight participants were randomly assigned to either the vegan diet group or to continue their usual diet. The impact of the diet intervention on hot flashes was assessed after 12 weeks. The results showed a significant impact of the vegan diet in improving the frequency and severity of hot flashes. Total hot flashes decreased by 79% and moderate-to-severe hot flashes decreased by 84% in the intervention group. At 12 weeks, most of the intervention-group participants reported no moderate-to-severe hot flashes at all. In addition, the vegan group showed improvements in measures of quality of life. It should be noted that, to a lesser degree, there were improvements in symptoms in the control group too. The authors state that possible reasons for benefit seen in the control group could include the natural decline in symptoms after menopause, the cooler temperatures approaching the study conclusion in December, or the control group participants' awareness of the vegan dietary intervention and their eagerness to implement it, despite being asked not to. In addition, the placebo effect of just being in a clinical trial cannot be underestimated.

There are good reasons why a healthy vegan diet with soya may be beneficial. Soya beans contain isoflavones, phyto-oestrogens which have previously been shown to reduce the incidence of hot flashes[16]. Isoflavones are converted to equol by gut bacteria, and higher production of equol, associated with better diet quality, has been associated with a lower frequency of hot flashes[17]. Previous studies have shown that vegetarians and vegans are better at producing equol than meat eaters[18]. The study discussed is of course small and of short duration, but the results are compelling given that conventional medical treatments for menopausal symptoms, such as hormone replacement therapy (HRT), come with side-effects and that a plant-based dietary pattern, including soya, significantly reduces the risk of the commonest causes of illness in older women – namely cardiovascular disease (CVD) and cancer. In fact, higher blood levels of equol may protect against cognitive decline with ageing[19].

12.7 Improvement in autoimmune diseases

Although the literature on this topic is less extensive, there are clear benefits of a plant-based diet, including a fully plant-based diet, in people with autoimmune diseases. This is a broad category of chronic conditions with a rising prevalence ranging from rheumatoid and psoriatic arthritis to lupus, inflammatory bowel disease and multiple sclerosis. A plant-based diet reduces inflammation, promotes a healthy immune system and optimises the health of the gut microbiome, all important for treating autoimmune conditions. This is due to the abundance of antioxidant and anti-inflammatory nutrients and fibre, whilst eliminating saturated fat and animal protein, known to have the opposite effects[17, 19, 20, 21].

Case reports and small studies have shown improvements in pain, quality of life, a reduced need for medications and in some cases elimination of medications entirely[23] in patients with autoimmune disease who have adopted a plant-based diet. There have even been reports of dramatic improvements, including remission of psoriatic arthritis[24] and Crohn's disease[25] and improvements in kidney function in lupus such that patients no longer required dialysis or a kidney transplant[26]. Regardless of whether a plant-based diet can reverse these diseases, it can be used alongside conventional medical treatments to improve outcomes and the effectiveness of the medications[27], whilst at the same time helping to reduce the elevated risk of CVD and cancer that occurs in people with autoimmune conditions[27, 28].

12.8 Prevention of migraines

An estimated 8% of Canadians[30] and 10% of the UK population suffer from migraines, with a significant impact on quality of life and productivity, and ranking as the sixth cause of disability in the world[31]. There is limited evidence of dietary interventions, other than eliminating known personal triggers (chocolate, cheese, citrus, alcohol, caffeine). There is some evidence for migraine prevention with riboflavin (vitamin B2), coenzyme Q10 (CoQ10), magnesium, butterbur root extract (*Petasites hybridus*), and feverfew (*Tanacetum parthenium*)[32]. One study suggested improvement in pain, frequency and duration with a low-fat diet[33].

What about a specifically plant-based diet? A randomised cross-over study looked at the effects of a low-fat plant-based diet intervention on migraine severity and frequency in 42 participants[34]. This 36-week study included two treatments, with 16 weeks for each treatment, which were (1) dietary instruction and (2) placebo supplement (a mixture of omega-3 oils and vitamin E), with a washout period of four weeks in between. During the diet intervention, participants were prescribed four weeks of a low-fat plant-based diet, then introduced an elimination diet of common triggers whilst continuing the low-fat plant-based diet. Significant decreases in reported pain, headache intensity, duration and percentage of headaches requiring pain relief medication were observed during the diet period compared with the placebo supplement, as well as reductions in body weight and total, LDL- and HDL-cholesterol. There are limitations to this study, including teasing out the effect of the elimination diet versus the low-fat plant-based diet, but this is certainly an area for further research and would be worth trialling on an individual basis for migraine sufferers.

12.9 Prevention of cataracts and age-related macular degeneration (AMD)

Cataracts form when protein builds up in the lens of the eye and makes it cloudy. Cataracts are very common, especially with ageing, and the main cause of impaired vision worldwide. Underlying conditions, medication and treatments can increase the risk, and this includes smoking, diabetes, steroid use, radiation, eye injuries and alcohol use. Two studies have shown that a plant-based diet can reduce the risk of cataracts.

In the Tzu Chi Health Study, which included over 6000 Buddhist volunteers, a vegetarian diet was associated with a 20% lower risk of developing cataracts during the almost six years of follow up[35]. These results are very similar to those published in 2011 from the EPIC-Oxford cohort in which there was a stepwise reduction in risk of cataracts as the amount of animal-derived foods in the diet decreased, with vegetarians and vegans having a 30% and 40% reduced risk respectively[36].

Why would this be? Vegetarian and vegan diets are associated with lower levels of inflammation and oxidative stress than meat-based diets. These diets are also higher in foods and nutrients associated with better eye health – carotenoids, vitamin C, folate, vitamin E and leafy greens – and much lower in harmful compounds found in animal foods: haem iron, heterocyclic amines and advanced glycation end products.

Another concern for ophthalmic health is age-related macular degeneration (AMD), the leading cause of irreversible central vision loss in developed countries. With the ageing population, AMD is set to become an increasing issue worldwide. Risk factors for developing AMD include lifestyle-related diseases and factors, such as smoking, hypertension, CVD, diabetes, a higher body mass index (BMI) and a high-fat diet. In contrast, a diet rich in fruit and vegetables and omega-3 fatty acids is associated with lower risk. Studies show higher fish or oily fish consumption to be associated with a lower risk of AMD as well[36, 37, 38]. Please see Chapter 5 for discussion of fish and the potential downsides.

12.10 Prevention of gallstone disease

Gallstone disease is common, with an estimated prevalence of 10–25% in Westernised countries, causing a significant health burden. It can be asymptomatic or associated with pain, infection and/or inflammation, and may require hospitalisation and a cholecystectomy – removal of the gallbladder. Eighty to 90% of gallstones are made of crystallised cholesterol. Risk factors for gallstone disease include greater age, being female, family history, obesity, rapid weight loss, lifestyle factors such as lack of physical activity, smoking and dietary factors, including saturated fat, trans fat, haem iron intake and lack of fibre [40, 41, 42, 43].

Studies on the impact of diet on the incidence of gallstone disease have shown mixed results, some showing no impact[44], some showing reduced incidence with a vegetarian diet pattern[45] and healthy dietary patterns [43,46], with one study suggesting that a vegetarian diet increases the risk of symptomatic gallstone disease[47].

The study that showed that symptomatic gallstone disease was increased in vegetarians was from the EPIC-Oxford study[47]. This study followed 49,652 adults, one-third of whom were vegetarian or vegan, for an average of 14 years. There was a significant association of increased BMI with risk of symptomatic gallstone disease. However, after adjusting for BMI, there remained a 22% increased risk of symptomatic gallstone disease in the vegetarians. The reason for this association is unclear.

Studies showing a benefit of healthy dietary patterns in reducing the incidence of gallstone disease include a 2019 study from Taiwan which prospectively followed 4839 participants (1403 vegetarians and 3436 non-vegetarians) for an average of six years[45]. After adjusting for other risk factors, including BMI, diabetes, physical activity and blood cholesterol, the study showed that, in women, being on a vegetarian diet was associated with a 48% decreased risk of symptomatic gallstone disease compared with a non-vegetarian diet, although not in men.

Another analysis, of the Health Professionals Follow-up Study (HPFS), a prospective cohort study of 43,635 male US health professionals, scored their diets based on adherence to three healthy dietary patterns, including the alternative Mediterranean, Alternate Healthy Eating Index (AHEI-2010), and Dietary Approaches to Stop Hypertension (DASH)[46]. These diet quality scores have in common the consumption of healthy plant foods whilst minimising animal products and processed food. The results showed that high adherence to these diet patterns was associated with a 35% lower risk of symptomatic gallstone disease.

Another prospective cohort analysis followed 60,768 women from the Nurses' Health Study and 40,744 men from the HPFS[43]. High adherence to the Alternate Healthy Eating Index 2010, as well as other lifestyle factors including maintaining a healthy body weight and keeping physically active, was associated with a reduced incidence of symptomatic gallstone disease.

Elevated BMI has consistently been shown to be a risk factor in the incidence of gallstone disease. We know that following a plant-based dietary pattern is helpful in maintaining a healthy weight (see section 1.8). Despite some conflicting results, the preponderance of evidence does support following a diet pattern which promotes healthy foods such as fruit, vegetables, fibre, legumes, whole grains and nuts, and which minimises unhealthful foods such as red meat, processed foods and sugary beverages, to reduce gallstone disease.

12.11 Financial saving in medical care

Throughout this book, we have documented the health benefits of a plant-based diet. So, does this translate into reduced reliance on healthcare systems and hence cost savings for the individual and wider society? In the Tzu Chi Taiwanese study cohort, vegetarians were found to have a lower incidence of outpatient visits, which translated into 13% lower outpatient expenditure and 15% lower total medical expenditure[48].

It is interesting to hypothesise the health economic impact of a plant-based diet on the UK's cash-strapped National Health Service. In 2018, spending on healthcare in the UK totalled £214.4 billion – approximately £3227 per person[49]. If everyone in the country shifted to a vegetarian diet, this could (using the 15% reduction as a guide) reduce healthcare expenditure by £32 billion.

Total health spending by the Canadian government in 2019 was $186.5 billion, accounting for 23.4% of total government spending, and represents the largest expense among provincial, territorial and local governments combined, accounting for nearly one-third of their total spending in 2019. This was equivalent to $4910 per Canadian. An additional 30% of total health spending comes from the private sector[50]. In 2019, total health expenditure was expected to be of the order of $264.4 billion, or $7068 per Canadian, with overall health expenditure representing 11.6% of Canada's gross domestic product. If the country shifted to a vegetarian diet, then at the 15% potential reduction, this would be a saving of nearly 40 billion dollars[51]. This provides some pause for thought.

12.12 The COVID-19 pandemic

On 11 March 2020, the World Health Organization characterised coronavirus disease, COVID-19, caused by severe acute respiratory syndrome coronavirus 2 (SARS-CoV-2), as a pandemic. As of 13 September 2021, COVID-19 has been confirmed in over 220 countries and territories. The virus has infected over 225.5 million people worldwide, and the number of deaths has reached over 4.6 million[52].

Underlying health conditions and COVID-19

It did not take long for healthcare professionals in the front-line of the pandemic response to observe that people with underlying chronic health conditions had a greater risk of developing severe COVID-19, requiring hospitalisation, intensive care treatment and ultimately dying. These underlying health conditions were noted to be associated with a number of modifiable risk factors and included overweight and obesity, CVD, cancer and type 2 diabetes. In the UK, more than 90% of those who died in the first wave of the pandemic had at least one underlying chronic condition[53]. In the US, 64% of the risk of hospitalisation from COVID-19 was attributable to four underlying health conditions: hypertension, heart failure, type 2 diabetes and obesity[54]. These conditions are intimately related to four modifiable lifestyle factors: tobacco smoking, excessive alcohol consumption, lack of physical activity and unhealthy diets.

Many of these underlying chronic conditions can be prevented and modified by adopting a healthy plant-based diet and lifestyle. It is important to note that there are also risk factors that cannot be modified, such as age and male sex, as well as some that cannot easily be modified in the short term but are equally important to address, including socioeconomic status and racial disparities.

Impact of diet on the immune system and the gut microbiome in COVID-19

Early on in the pandemic, many clinicians and researchers began to write about the benefits of a healthy diet for supporting the immune system and improving our defences against the pandemic virus[55]. Most of this advice was empirical and based on evidence from other respiratory infections in which bioactive compounds found in fruit, vegetables, herbs and spices, such as vitamin C, flavonoids, carotenoids and curcumin, were associated with reduced severity and better outcomes. In addition, it was hypothesised that a healthier gut microbiome, given our knowledge of the gut-lung axis and its involvement in mounting a robust immune response, may be important[56].

We now have a scientific basis from which to make these recommendations. A study from China analysed the composition of the gut microbiome and measured blood markers of in-flammation in 100 hospitalised patients with COVID-19 and compared the results with samples taken from 78 healthy volunteers[57]. Serial stool samples were collected from 27 of the 100 patients up to 30 days after clearance of SARS-CoV-2. Patients with COVID-19 had significant alterations in the composition of the gut microbiome, compared with people without the infection, including reductions in bacterial species that are known to regulate the immune response. These strains of bacteria thrive on dietary fibre and are important in producing short-chain fatty acids, which reduce inflammation and regulate the immune system. In addition, these alterations were more pronounced in patients with a severe disease course and were associated with higher levels of inflammatory markers in the blood.

It is worth remembering that the American Gut Project, one of the largest studies to evaluate the human gut microbiome, has observed that people consuming more than 30 different types of plant foods a week have a healthier and more diverse gut microbiome than people consuming fewer than 10 different plant types[58].

Diet patterns and COVID-19

The first publication to highlight the importance of a healthy plant-based diet pattern reported the results of a case-control study of healthcare workers, mostly physicians, with significant exposure to COVID-19 patients from six countries[59]. Participants completed a web-based survey from 17 July to 25 September 2020. Information was collected on basic demographic characteristics, past medical history, medications, lifestyle and COVID-19 symptoms, and a 47-item food frequency questionnaire. The questions captured the dietary patterns of participants over the prior one year and included 11 choices: whole foods, plant-based diet; keto diet; vegetarian diet; Mediterranean diet; pescatarian diet; Palaeolithic diet; low-fat diet; low-carbohydrate diet; high-protein diet; other; none of the above. For the analysis, 'whole foods, plant-based' diets and 'vegetarian' diets were placed into one category called 'plant-based diets' (n=254). For the pescatarian diet, data were combined from those following a whole-foods plant-based, vegetarian and pescatarian diet, the latter only being 40 participants (n=294). The study included 568 people with COVID-19 and 2316 controls. Those participants who had had COVID-19 were asked to rate the severity of their symptoms based on five options from very mild to critical, requiring intensive care.

The results showed that those following a plant-based diet pattern had a 73% reduction in the risk of moderate or severe COVID-19 and those following a pescatarian diet had a 59% reduction in risk. This was independent of BMI and underlying chronic health conditions. In contrast, participants following a high-protein, low-carbohydrate diet had a three-fold higher risk of moderate or severe COVID-19 when compared with the plant-based group.

This was not a study of people following a vegan or 100% plant-based diet, despite the media headlines suggesting the contrary. In fact, those classified as plant-based were not that healthy, consuming a median of 3.7 portions of legumes and 9.8 portions of fruit per week and still consuming some animal foods, including similar amounts of dairy and eggs to the non-plant-based group, and similar amounts of refined grains. However, their consumption of legumes, nuts and vegetables was significantly higher and consumption of red/processed meat, sugar-sweetened beverages and alcohol significantly lower than those participants who did not follow a plant-based diet.

The second paper published reported more robust data from the now well-publicised Zoe COVID symptom study[60]. This paper analysed diet quality in more than half a million participants from the US and UK. During the follow-up period, 31,815 COVID-19 cases were documented. Adherence to a healthy plant-based diet was calculated using the healthy plant-based diet index which gives positive marks to healthy plant foods, and negative marks to unhealthy plant foods and all animal foods. Those eating a healthy plant-based diet had a 10% reduction in risk of getting COVID-19 and a 40% reduction in the risk of getting severe disease. The impact of a healthy diet was greatest in those from lower socioeconomic groups and independent of underlying chronic health conditions, BMI, smoking and physical activity. Based on these results, it was calculated that nearly a third of COVID-19 cases could have been prevented if these differences in diet quality and wealth had not existed.

There are limitations to this study. It is observational, with self-selected participants, self-reported dietary information and, for the primary outcome of COVID-19 infection, a validated symptom-based algorithm was used rather than PCR test results. However, this is likely to be the best evidence we can expect to have outside of a randomised study. The authors concluded:

'Our data provide evidence that a healthy diet was associated with lower risk of COVID-19 and severe COVID-19 even after accounting for other healthy behaviors, social determinants of health, and virus transmission measures.'

'Long-COVID' and diet

Many patients infected with SARS-CoV-2 continue to experience symptoms after the acute phase of infection, including fatigue, sleep difficulties, anxiety and depression, shortness of breath, hair loss, arthralgia and muscle weakness[61]. The term 'long-COVID' has been coined for this post-COVID -19 syndrome, which is associated with signs and symptoms that may last weeks to months and impose a substantial burden on affected individuals. Whether a plant-based diet might be useful to alleviate some symptoms related to long-COVID has not yet been examined in clinical trials. However, we do know from pre-pandemic studies that a plant-based dietary pattern may be of general benefit for some symptoms that are seen with long COVID-19, including fatigue, sleep disorders, headaches, anxiety, depression and musculoskeletal pain, and we believe it should be one of the strategies, including other lifestyle measures, to help improve the quality of life and symptoms of those suffering from long-COVID[62].

Conclusion

Based on the available evidence, we can say that any shift to a more plant-based way of eating will improve health outcomes during and beyond the current pandemic. Systematic national and international efforts to promote plant-based eating and other healthful lifestyle measures will help to address the current pandemic of chronic non-communicable diseases and build resilience for the current COVID-19 pandemic as well as future ones that are surely to come.

Chapter 13

Considerations for planetary health

13.1 How does my diet choice impact the climate and ecological crises?

The global food system is a direct driver of three inter-related global crises: nutrition, climate and ecological. We have covered extensively the impact of our diet choices on personal health but our diet choice also has an enormous impact on planetary health[1].

Greenhouse gases and climate change

Greenhouse gas (GHG) emissions are contributing significantly to global warming and climate change. The Intergovernmental Panel on Climate Change (IPCC) has warned us about the dire consequences of the projected global warming of 1.5°C above pre-industrial levels, which could happen in the next decade. This includes extreme heat, increased and more frequent flooding and droughts, rising sea levels, species loss and extinction, and risks to human health, livelihoods, food security, water supply and economic growth. Their most recent (6th) IPCC Report, released in 2021, states that it is 'unequivocal' that human activity has warmed the atmosphere, the ocean and the land on a scale that is 'unprecedented' over thousands of years[2]. Already human-induced climate change is resulting in many weather and climate extremes in every region across the globe. Many changes due to GHG emissions are already 'irreversible' for centuries to millennia. GHG concentrations have continued to increase and are 'attributed largely to human activities, mostly fossil fuel use, land use change and agriculture'. Urgent action is needed.

The goal of the Paris Agreement is to prevent this catastrophic rise in temperature, yet, in 2020, scientists warned that without a drastic change to our food system, we will not be able to keep within these temperature limits and that dietary change is *the* most important approach to meeting these climate-change targets[3, 4, 5].

Half of the world's habitable land is used for agriculture with more than 80% of farmland globally used for meat and dairy farming, be it for grazing animals or growing food for animals. Even though estimates vary, the food system is responsible for over a quarter, if not a third, of the world's GHG emissions and the production and consumption of meat, dairy and eggs accounts for more than 60% of these emissions[2, 3].

A more recent paper presented the results of a Global Sensitivity Analysis and suggested that animal agriculture is in fact responsible for a whopping 87% of GHG emissions[8]. Even the most sustainably produced animal foods generate more GHG emissions than any plant foods, regardless of the distance travelled to get to your plate[1]. The emissions from animal agriculture are greater than those from all forms of transportation combined.

It is not just the carbon emissions from animal agriculture which are problematic but also methane produced by wetland rice systems and ruminant animals, and nitrous oxide from fertiliser and manure. Methane is an even more potent GHG than carbon, by 25 times, trapping the sun's heat and warming the earth 86 times as much as the same mass of carbon dioxide over a 20-year period. Within animal farming, methane is generated from the burps of ruminant animals – principally, cows and sheep – and global emissions continue to rise dramatically, in part due to animal agriculture and farming[9]. Raising ruminant animals for meat and dairy alone accounts for around half the GHG emissions from animal agriculture[1].

Some argue that because methane is relatively short-lived in the atmosphere – only 10 years compared with hundreds of years for carbon dioxide – it matters less. This does not mean we should continue producing methane. It means we have a chance in a shorter period to significantly reduce these emissions. In fact, it seems we have been vastly underestimating the contribution of methane from intensively raised animals to GHG emissions by as much as 90% despite the prevailing narrative that factory farms use less land and are a more 'efficient' way to raise animals for food[10]. The United Nations is clear: we have to address methane emissions now in order to keep global warming below levels associated with irreversible and catastrophic consequences[11].

Nitrogen emissions from animal farming are also increasingly problematic[12]. These emissions come from nitrogen present in synthetic and organic fertilisers and animal manure and urine, resulting in nitrous oxide generation, another potent GHG gas. Nitrous oxide is 300 times more potent than carbon dioxide, trapping more heat and remaining in the atmosphere for longer than methane – over 100 years. Animal agriculture contributes around a third of nitrogen emissions, with most of that coming from the production of animal feed.

Pollution of our environment

The vast quantities of animal manure produced from farming not only emit nitrous oxide, but also contaminate land and pollute our water systems[13]. The safe management and disposal of this manure are becoming impossible tasks[14].

The waste from animal farming is contributing to air pollution from gases such as ammonia, hydrogen sulphide, nitrous oxide and methane. These gases have an adverse impact on human health, with farm workers and people living close to animal farming operations having an increased risk of asthma and other lung problems[15] and cardiovascular diseases[16]. A first-of-a-kind study from the US determined how the production of various foods impacted air quality and consequent health outcomes. The study showed that 17,900 deaths a year were attributable to air pollution caused by agriculture, with ammonia emissions, farm animal waste and fertiliser application accounting for most of these deaths. Altogether, 80% of these deaths were attributed to the production of animal-derived foods, with red meat the greatest contributor[17]. The production of all plant foods considered was less polluting than any animal foods. The authors concluded that a shift to vegetarian and vegan diets would vastly improve air-quality-related health issues.

What would be the impact of adopting a plant-based diet?

There is a vast inefficiency in the current food system when you consider that animal farming produces only 18% of the calories and 37% of the protein consumed globally while using over 80% of farmland[1]. Farmed animals themselves also consume more calories and protein than they produce for human consumption. Conservative estimates show that farmed animals consume between 6 and 12.5 kilograms of plant protein to produce a single kilogram of animal protein. This means that we currently produce enough food to feed two planets. If we were all to transition to eating a meat-rich diet typical of the 20 most industrialised countries, we would need seven planets to produce enough food[18].

If we all adopted a 100% plant-based or vegan diet we could reduce the land used for food production by 76%, and GHG emissions from the food system by up to 50%[1]. The land released would then be able to be used to capture significant amounts of carbon[19]. Crops can also be produced in a manner which allows for carbon sequestration into the soil instead of contributing to emissions, with further reductions in fossil fuel use also possible[20]. Further studies have examined the impact of shifting towards plant-based diets on both human and environmental health and concluded definitively that it would provide combined benefits[21]. Plant-based diets could reduce GHG emissions by 56% and other environmental impacts of the food system by 6-22%, whilst at the same time improving the nutritional quality of our diet, significantly reducing the burden of chronic disease and reducing premature mortality by 22%. When considering protein sources, tofu, beans, nuts and peas have the lowest carbon footprint compared with any source of animal protein and their consumption has significant advantages for human health[1].

Wildlife and biodiversity loss

Although we often focus on GHG emissions, the global food system, particularly animal agriculture, has a far broader impact on planetary health. Animal agriculture is the biggest driver of wildlife and biodiversity loss, species extinction, land use change and land degradation, deforestation, freshwater use, water pollution and ocean destruction[22]. Through our actions we have wiped out 60% of wildlife populations since 1970 and have now entered what is termed the 'sixth mass extinction event' where an estimated one million animal and plant species are threatened with extinction[23].

Land use change, mainly land conversion for crop production, raising farmed animals and plantations, is the strongest driver of our destruction of nature[22]. It is estimated that around 60% of wildlife loss is related to agriculture and the industrial methods we use[24]. Nearly 90% of our ecosystems, both terrestrial and marine, are degraded or severely degraded, while only 11% are estimated to be in reasonable condition[25]. The terrible impact of climate change and ecosystem destruction on our planetary life support systems has led to an unprecedented existential threat to the survival of the human species. Yet one major solution is clear and in our collective control: a global shift to a plant-based food system[26].

13.2 Is raising grass-fed animals or organic meat better for the environment?

The counter-arguments to reducing and eliminating the consumption of animal foods are commonplace. Many continue to suggest that raising grass-fed animals for food rather than intensively raised factory-farmed animals could be part of the climate solution by helping to reduce GHG emissions. This assumes that grazing animals can contribute to regenerating farmland and increasing the potential for that land to act as a carbon store. This would then partially or completely offset the GHG emissions generated. However, most research to date has shown that this type of animal agriculture would continue to be a net emitter of GHGs and, in fact, methane generation is greater when animals consume grass rather than grain. In addition, it is likely that an equilibrium will eventually be reached between the carbon being produced and that which can be stored in the soil, and therefore the land can no longer contribute to removal of carbon from the atmosphere. The level of carbon saturation depends on the particular ecosystem, but every ecosystem has a limit after which no more carbon can be stored.

This type of animal farming system also uses much more land than raising animals in factory operations and certainly could not support anywhere close to the current levels of global meat consumption[27].

Clearing land to graze ruminant animals is a major driver of deforestation and loss of biodiversity and this change in land use further contributes to the GHG emissions of animal agriculture. That same land could be used instead to store carbon through the planting of trees or conserving and restoring nature[27].

Another factor is that grass-fed cows take much longer to get to slaughter weight and therefore more cows would be needed to meet the current global demand if we relied on these animals. A modelling study from the US showed that, if everyone shifted to consuming only grass-fed beef, 30% more cows would be needed to meet demand yet the current land available could only supply at best 60% of the demand[28]. Organic meat production has also been modelled to be vastly more damaging to the environment than plant-based food sources[29]. Overall, it is estimated that changes in food production practices could reduce agricultural GHG emissions in 2050 by about 10%, whereas increased consumption of plant-based diets could reduce emissions by up to 80%. A further 5% reduction could be achieved by halving food loss and waste[30].

Given that animal farming is a major contributor to the loss of animal and plant biodiversity[31], studies have shown that preserving and restoring nature and protecting wetlands and woodlands would have greater economic benefits to people and society than using the land to grow food. For many reasons it's clear that reducing animal grazing is required, which means a vast knock-on reduction in consumption of animal foods[32].

13.3 Don't you need animals to nourish the soil?

Our current predominantly tillage-based crop agriculture is not fit for purpose and is causing widespread soil and environmental degradation. This has led to higher production costs, lower farm productivity and profit, suboptimal yield ceilings and poor efficiency and resilience, and is not climate smart. These facts are widely accepted, but the proposed solutions differ, with many suggesting that animal grazing and manure are a required element for restoring soil health[32, 33].

Animal manure is a source of nitrogen, a nutrient that is required for growing plants. When animals eat plants some of the nitrogen is recycled back to the soil through their faeces and urine, thus delivering nutrients back to the soil for further growth of plants. However, much of the nitrogen from faeces remains in the soil and is converted to nitrous oxide or other chemical forms that result in land, air and water pollution. Yet, nitrogen is ubiquitous in the atmosphere and some plants, such as legumes, and bacteria in the soil can draw nitrogen out of the atmosphere into the soil. In addition, earthworms present in healthy soil can recycle nutrients by digesting plant biomass and adding nitrogen and other nutrients back into the soil. There is absolutely no need to use ruminant animals as an intermediary for this process[35].

The solutions to many of our current problems in crop agriculture are provided by no-till Conservation Agriculture, which is an ecosystem approach to regenerative and sustainable agriculture based upon the context-specific application of three interlinked principles of ecological sustainability and resilience[36]:

1. Continuous no- or minimum-mechanical soil disturbance, by seeding or planting directly into untilled soil, and no-till weeding.
2. Maintaining permanent biomass mulch cover on the soil surface using crop biomass stubbles and cover crops to protect and feed soil life.
3. Diversifying species – both annuals and perennials – with rotations, sequences and associations.

These universally applicable core principles go hand in hand with other complementary good agricultural practices, including integrated crop, soil, nutrient, water, pest and energy management.

'Conservation Agriculture' describes a combination of resource-conserving practices simultaneously creating synergies between them to regenerate soil and landscape health, and functions to optimise sustainable production. It does not require any inputs from farmed animals as the healthy soil and its components are self-sustaining without the need for animal grazing and manure. Conservation Agriculture promotes soil health by improving soil organic matter content, soil structure, soil moisture and nutrient-holding capacity. Soil meso-fauna and a range of soil micro-organisms help to biologically incorporate organic matter into the soil. Earthworms in particular are able to ingest biomass high in lignin and cellulose, combining it with soil mineral particles in their guts and producing worm casts that are rich in plant nutrients. Fungi also help to sequester carbon and convert it into a more stable form which helps to create soil aggregates and increase soil porosity that in turn enhances water infiltration and retention and soil aeration.

Conservation Agriculture requires much smaller inputs of chemicals and fossil fuel than tillage-based agriculture and it is entirely possible to practise it within organic farming systems with biological forms of integrated pest management. It offers many productivity, economic, environmental and social benefits, including higher and stable production and profit; control of run-off, erosion and land degradation; greater quantities of clean water; enhanced climate change adaptability and mitigation; improved water cycling and reduced risks of flooding; and rehabilitation of degraded lands, biodiversity and ecosystem functions[35, 36, 37].

13.4 I have heard that rice farming also produces GHGs?

Many will point out that rice farming is also an emitter of both methane and nitrous oxide, and with rice being a staple food for nearly half the world's population, action is required to mitigate against these emissions. This is true for wetland rice systems in which anaerobic soil conditions lead to methane production. Rice farming contributes 2.5% of global GHG emissions from agriculture and 15-20% of the total methane emissions from human activities, whereas nitrous oxide emissions are not as rigorously reported[39]. However, methane is generated because of the predominant farming practices of flooding rice paddies and growing rice in anaerobic conditions in which methane is produced by fermenting anaerobic bacteria. There are readily available solutions with farming methods that greatly reduce the production of methane from rice fields. For example, no-till rice production systems under aerobic soil conditions, as in Conservation Agriculture systems, significantly reduce methane and nitrous oxide production, and water, fertiliser and fuel use.

The System of Rice Intensification (SRI) is a climate-smart way of farming rice that increases productivity whilst significantly reducing inputs. Irrigation water is reduced by 30-50% and chemical fertiliser by 20-100%, with reduced need for pesticides too[40]. Aeration of the soil reduces the production of methane by up to 60%.

Even though the criticism of methods such as SRI include the fact that nitrous oxide emissions can increase due to their production by aerobic microbes in the soil, the net reduction in GHG emissions is of the order of 40%[40, 41]. Of course, further work is needed to reduce these GHG emissions, but it does not provide an excuse to continue the consumption of meat and dairy, which makes by far the greater contribution to global emissions.

Diversifying the plant foods in our diet is also part of the solution. Currently rice, maize and wheat contribute 60% of the calories consumed by humans[30]. There are many underused grains that have excellent nutritional profiles and can have advantages for climate health. These include quinoa, millet, amaranth, sorghum and teff.

13.5 What about water use? I have heard that it takes a lot of water to produce almond milk?

The agricultural sector uses 70% of the freshwater available worldwide, while the production of animal-based products accounts for almost one third of that water use[43]. The question of almonds has come about due to the amount of water used for irrigation in growing almonds, particularly in California. It certainly can use a lot of water, but even then, almond milk is less water-intensive than the production of cow's milk and, in addition, requires significantly less land use and produces fewer GHG emissions. It takes about 371 litres of water to produce 1 litre of almond milk. By comparison, it can take up to 628 litres of water to produce 1 litre of dairy milk. Oat milk and soya milk have the lowest water use, with oat milk using 48 litres and soya milk 28 litres to produce 1 litre[1, 43]. If you are concerned about the water use then we would suggest avoiding almonds or almond milk sourced from California.

13.6 Is eating fish more sustainable than eating meat?

When you consider that over 90% of global wild fish stocks have been overfished or fished at capacity, then advocating for fish to be included in the diet of nearly eight billion people on this planet does not make sense from a sustainability perspective[45]. Fishing is damaging ocean habitats through overexploitation, by-catch of non-target species, seafloor habitat destruction from sea floor trawling, illegal and unreported fishing, dumped fishing gear and completely changing natural biodiversity, with the potential for irreversible long-term consequences for planetary health.

There are, of course, small communities in low-income countries that rely on fisheries for their food and livelihood.

These communities may have to continue with this industry until alternative sources of food and income can be generated. For most humans on this planet, eating fish is not necessary and is certainly not sustainable. Fish obtain long-chain omega-3 fatty acids from marine algae and so can humans. We should invest in companies that are finding more novel and sustainable ways of producing healthy nutrients, and algae are increasingly being recognised as a good alternative source[46].

Marine plastic pollution

We are all concerned about the level of plastic pollution in our oceans. It is estimated that up to 12 million tonnes of plastic end up in the oceans every year, most of it starting out on land. However, it is often forgotten that at least 10% of this plastic comes from the fishing industry, from abandoned fishing equipment, with some estimates as high as 46%. Fishing equipment also contributes to large plastics found floating at the surface, with additional rubbish from the industry, such as packing containers, tape and buoys also adding further to this plastics pollution[46, 47]. The abandoned fishing gear continues to trap and kill sea animals, and the plastic pollution is hazardous to all sea life. There are increasing concerns that exposure to microplastics in our food chain may be a health concern for humans too[48, 49].

Aquaculture (farmed fish)

The fish in aquafarms are kept in cramped and dirty conditions, causing diseases, injuries and death in the fish. This necessitates the use of antibiotics, pesticides and other chemicals. Waste from the aquafarms, including faeces, uneaten food and the chemicals used, pollute the surrounding ocean and coastal areas and cause destruction of marine life and natural habitats.

Farmed fish infected with diseases or parasites can spread these to their wild counterparts, affecting the health of wild populations near fish farms. Farming carnivorous species requires large inputs of fish-feed composed largely of fishmeal and fish oil made from wild-caught fish, hardly contributing to sustainability when over 90% of global wild fish stocks have been overfished or fished at capacity.

13.7 Surely, if we don't eat meat then world hunger will increase?

One in nine people on this planet suffer from hunger, yet we produce enough food to feed at least 10 billion people[50, 51]. Independent analysis suggests that the true figure for those suffering from hunger may in fact be much higher than the official UN figures and that around two billion people remain hungry[53].

The trouble is that our food system is inefficient and wasteful. For example, 41% of crops grown globally that could be eaten by humans are fed to farmed animals; however, animal-based foods only provide 18% of global calories and 37% of protein. On average, 12.5 kilograms of plant protein fed to farmed animals produces just 1 kilogram of animal protein[1]. The conversion efficiency ratio varies based on different animals[54]. For example, 25 kilograms of animal feed is required to produce 1 kilogram of beef, whereas 3.3 kilograms of feed will produce 1 kilogram of chicken. Only 1.9% of calories fed to cattle are converted to calories for humans; the remaining 98.1% are lost during conversion. For poultry, 13% of calories are converted to calories for humans. World hunger could be eradicated if we just used food crops for humans rather than animals.

These figures do not even take into consideration food waste. One-third of food produced for human consumption is wasted somewhere along the supply chain, amounting to about 1.3 billion tons per year[54, 55]. More than 50% of this waste in Europe and North America occurs in our own homes, with animal-derived foods spoiling and thus being wasted more often.

When considering the food we need to consume for health, global meat consumption exceeds recommended levels by 20% yet fruit and vegetable consumption is 38% below healthy minimum levels. The situation is worse still in North America and Europe. Meat and dairy consumption increases with wealth, and to meet healthy eating guidelines, meat consumption would need to be reduced by at least 50%, if not up to 90%, and fruit and vegetable consumption increased by 100%[29, 56]. This needs to be matched on the production side. The growing demand for meat is not only contributing to environmental destruction but is also compounding world hunger. Yet modelling studies show that replacing beef, pork, dairy, poultry and eggs with plant-based foods would allow a 2-to-20-fold increase in the production of nutritionally similar plant foods, with removal of beef, dairy and pork having a greater impact than removing poultry and eggs. For the US alone, it is estimated that a fully plant-based food system could therefore feed an extra 350 million people[58].

13.8 Even if we stop animal agriculture, I have heard the land freed up is not suitable for growing crops?

A global shift to a plant-based food system would free up 75% or more of agricultural land that is currently used for animal pasture and to grow crops to feed animals, whilst still being able to produce enough food for the global population[1]. This land could instead be allowed to re-wild, restore natural habitats and biodiversity and act as a store of carbon[19]. Meanwhile, the crops that are used to feed animals can instead be used as food for humans. Countries that import grain for human consumption could start growing their own and become self-reliant.

If you consider that most of the soya grown on land cleared in the Amazon is fed to farmed animals and not humans, you can appreciate how much land would become available. Deforestation of the Amazon is expanding not only to grow feed but to graze animals to meet the increasing global demand of consumers for meat[59]. This is just one example of loss of natural habitats that is taking place around the world.

The continued human destruction and encroachment on wildlife habitats is accelerating us into the sixth mass extinction event. A rather alarming study has estimated that over the entire 20th century more than 500 land vertebrate species have become extinct, but that the same number again could become extinct in the next two decades[23]. It is human activities such as the wildlife trade and animal farming that are driving the extinction of animals and changing our ecosystems, factors which are already resulting in devastating consequences for human survival and health. To return pasture and cropland to their natural form would go a long way to restoring the balance of our planet. In fact, the benefit of restoring nature is much greater for people and society than using that land for grazing animals or growing food[32].

13.9 If we all switch from dairy milk to soya milk, won't this worsen the destruction of the Amazon?

The media love to suggest that the rising number of vegans are responsible for deforestation of the Amazon. Nothing could be further from the truth. More than 70% of soya grown in the Amazon is used to feed farmed animals[1]. The rest is used for biofuels, industry or vegetable oils. Only around 7% of all soya grown globally is used in foods such as soya milk, cheese and yoghurt, and tofu and tempeh. There has been an exponential increase in the production of soya, especially in US and Brazil, where most of the world's soya is produced. This is driven by the demand for animal feed, biofuels and vegetable oils. Yet despite this increased production, the main driver of Amazon deforestation remains clearing land for grazing animals and not soya production[60]. The 2% of soya that is used to make soya milk is not sourced from the Amazon. Countries mainly source this non-genetically modified soya from Europe, US and China. So, there is little risk that soya grown in the Amazon is ending up in your soya drink.

The most comprehensive analysis of the environmental impact of the food system showed that the production of 1 litre of cow's milk requires more than 22 times more water and 12 times more land than 1 litre of soya milk, whilst generating three times more GHG emissions[1].

13.10 But infections have been transmitted by eating spinach?

The only reason that plant foods such as spinach, cucumber and salad leaves become contaminated with bacteria is through exposure to animal manure or contaminated water used for irrigation, or if these foods come into contact with bacteria during the food processing stage. Plant foods are very rarely a direct source of infection. Food-borne infections, predominantly caused by bacteria such as *Staphylococcus aureus, Salmonella* species, *Campylobacter* species, *Listeria monocytogenes*, and *E. coli*, are essentially zoonotic diseases and associated with consumption of infected animal products or plant foods that have been contaminated somewhere along the food chain[60, 61].

One of the most comprehensive studies of the worldwide burden of food-borne illnesses estimated that in 2010 there were 582 million cases of infection caused by contaminated food, with 351,000 deaths[63]. In 2018, there were nearly 50,000 cases of foodborne infection in the European Union with one in three cases caused by *Salmonella*, mainly linked to the consumption of eggs[64]. In Canada, there are around four million cases of food poisoning every year. The commonest infections are *Norovirus* from shellfish, *Salmonella* and *Campylobacter* from chicken and eggs and *E. coli* in faeces from a variety of animals[65].

13.11 What has antibiotic resistance got to do with my diet choice?

Another major issue with our current food system, which threatens global health, is the widespread use of antibiotics in animal agriculture. Around 40–70% of all antibiotics globally are sold for use in animals and it has been recognised for many years that agricultural use of antibiotics is a major contributor to antibiotic-resistant infections in humans[66]. We are entering a post-antibiotic era where it is no longer unusual to be treating patients who have infections for which there are no suitable antibiotics.

A 2016 review of antibiotic resistance commissioned by the UK Prime Minister suggested that, globally, 700,000 lives are lost annually from antibiotic-resistant infections and by 2050 this number could be as high as 10 million[67]. One of the 10 recommendations in the report was the reduction of antibiotic use in animal agriculture. However, with the increasing industrialisation of food production and the growing demand for meat, this will be impossible to achieve without governments working together. This is a global issue which requires a global solution and reducing antibiotic-resistant organisms in our food system needs to be a priority.

The issues that arise from using antibiotics in animal farming are that animals then carry antibiotic-resistant strains of common bacteria such as *E coli* and *Salmonella* species. These strains can be transmitted between animals, can contaminate the surrounding environment and soil leading to contamination of plant food crops, and can be transmitted to humans directly from the consumption of the animals, from contaminated plant foods or to those working in slaughter houses[67, 68]. Humans are also exposed to antibiotic residues from farming waste through exposure to manure and contaminated soil and water systems[70]. This low-level exposure also selects for carriage of antibiotic-resistant strains of bacteria in humans and adversely impacts the health of the gut microbiome. Interestingly, some studies that have examined the gut bacteria of those consuming different types of diet have shown that vegans have a lower prevalence of bacteria with antibiotic-resistance genes compared with people consuming an omnivorous or vegetarian diet. This suggests that exposure to animal foods is a risk factor for carriage of antibiotic-resistant bacteria[70, 71, 72].

Sadly, you rarely hear the reduction or elimination of meat consumption recommended as a necessary solution to this serious problem, yet one analysis found that if we all limited meat consumption to 40 grams per day – the equivalent of one standard fast-food burger per person – we could reduce the global use of antibiotics in animals raised for food by 66%[74].

13.12 Why is eating animals linked to pandemics?

Industrialisation of animal farming, along with the wildlife trade and habitat destruction, has led to the perfect conditions necessary for the transmission of novel infections, mostly viruses, from animals to humans ('zoonoses') with epidemic and pandemic potential. Several zoonotic pandemics that have occurred in the last century can be traced back to our farming practices and the use of animals as food[74, 75]. In fact, three out of four new and emerging infections are zoonoses – that is, arise in animals and then jump to humans.

Studies have shown that there is a direct association between the increase in animal farming, the loss of biodiversity and the increasing threat of zoonotic infections. The conversion of wild habitats to farmland destroys the natural ecosystems and wipes out larger species, leaving behind smaller animals, such as rats and bats, which are more likely to carry infections that can be passed on to humans[77]. These smaller animals are mobile and adaptable and can produce lots of offspring rapidly.

In addition, the increasing industrialisation of animal agriculture means that most farmed animals are raised on factory farms, kept in cramped and squalid conditions, suffer from stress and disease and thus are more likely to succumb to infections. These infections can be passed on to other animals, mutate and eventually have the potential to be passed on to humans[77, 78, 79]. In the UK and Canada, more than 70% of animals raised for food are kept on factory farms, 99% in the US and 90% worldwide[81].

An even bigger threat than coronavirus for causing a future pandemic is a bird flu. Recent strains include H5N1, which was first detected in humans in 1997, causing a major outbreak in 2004, and H7N9, which was first detected in 2013. Both originated in wild birds and were transmitted to humans via poultry farming. Although transmission to humans is currently rare, when it does occur there is a 60% chance of dying from H5N1 and about 30% from H7N9[81, 82]. It is only a matter of time before these viruses adapt and become more transmissible to humans and, when they do, the results could be catastrophic. In fact, it is already happening. In February 2021, the media reported the first case of H5N8 bird flu in humans[84]. Many of us consider the COVID-19 pandemic a warning with worse in store if farming practices do not change.

Chapter 14

Final thoughts

14.1 What is the most important health question to ask about your diet?

The most important question to ask of your diet is: 'Will it provide protection against heart disease and cancer?' These are the top two killers of men and women around the globe. The good news is that a diet focused around or exclusively on whole plant foods is associated with the lowest risks of both heart disease and cancer. The same cannot be said for any other diet pattern. Before you jump onto the latest fad diet bandwagon, ask whether this diet has decades of scientific evidence supporting the prevention and potential reversal of chronic illness. If the answer is no, then it's not worth the risk.

The simple truth about a healthy diet is not going to change anytime soon. We know enough now to say that if you centre your diet on fruit, vegetables, whole grains, legumes, nuts and seeds, you will have the best chance of avoiding chronic illness and living a longer life in good health.

In addition to cardiovascular disease (CVD) and cancer, there is a global pandemic of overweight and obesity and type 2 diabetes. These chronic conditions together are contributing to the rising burden of dementia. We are also increasingly spending more than a decade in ill health before we die[1]. In fact, in some high-income countries, such as the UK and US, life-expectancy has started to slow and decline for the first time in history[2, 3]. This book has highlighted the immense power of a plant-based diet not only to prevent these chronic conditions but to halt their progression, and to reverse them in some cases.

The benefits of a plant-predominant diet have made it into most national and international guidelines for prevention of chronic illness. This includes the American College of Cardiology's 2019 guidelines on prevention of CVD[4], the World Cancer Research Guidelines on cancer prevention[5] and the American College of Lifestyle Medicine's position statement on type 2 diabetes[6].

14.2 What lies behind the growth of the Lifestyle Medicine movement?

As you now know from reading this book, according to the Global Burden of Disease Study of 195 countries, dietary factors are the single leading cause of death globally, an even greater health burden than smoking[7]. Despite this, nutrition education is not a standard part of medical training; at most it occupies a few hours in the whole medical curriculum. This was certainly the case for both of us. We came across the vast body of evidence on plant-based nutrition many years after we had qualified as physicians and after we had completed our specialty training. As a result, physicians remain unaware of the literature, and feel uncomfortable in educating their patients[8]. A systematic review in 2019 of medical nutrition education found that, despite wanting to receive nutrition education, graduating medical students are not adequately supported to provide high-quality, effective nutrition care to patients[9].

In recent years, we have seen an increasing number of nutrition education courses for healthcare professionals and also a growing movement of healthcare professionals from different disciplines and specialities, who recognise the importance of, and are gaining expertise in, the evidence-based field of Lifestyle Medicine. Lifestyle Medicine uses whole food, plant-predominant nutrition, and other important lifestyle measures of optimal sleep, physical activity, avoidance of risky substances such as tobacco and alcohol, social connection and stress management, as a primary preventative and treatment modality for chronic disease, where equal focus is placed on lifestyle medicine as on medications and procedures[10].

The benefit of Lifestyle Medicine is that it addresses the root cause of disease in order to improve health and allows us as individuals to take control of our own wellbeing. Lifestyle Medicine is now one of the fastest growing healthcare fields globally, recognised in the peer-reviewed literature, with the American College of Lifestyle Medicine as its flagship organisation[11]. We certainly view this progress with feelings of hope for a better way forward.

14.3 So, now you have decided to switch to a plant-based diet, what are the basics?

Our top tip is to 'always be prepared'. By this we mean that it is best to plan ahead, whether that is for your meals at home, your lunches at work, going to friends' houses or out to a restaurant. Although plant-based options have significantly increased over the last decade, you can't always guarantee a healthy plant-based meal or snack when you are out and about. Always carry some healthy snacks with you, such as fruit or some nuts and seeds. Call ahead when going out for a meal or try to select a restaurant with suitable options.

Here is some useful advice to start you on your journey[12]:

1. Aim to eat 10 portions of fruit and vegetables a day, focusing on all the colours of the rainbow. Five-a-day is just not enough. This can be a combination of frozen, tinned or fresh, with a mixture of raw and cooked. Try

to eat cruciferous vegetables, leafy greens and berries on most days.

2. Don't skip breakfast. Make oats your breakfast of choice. An easy way to save time in the morning is to soak oats overnight in your favourite calcium-fortified plant milk, keeping it in the fridge, so it's ready to eat first thing in the morning. Adding a portion of fruit and flaxseeds to your oats is a great way to increase the nutritional value of your breakfast.

3. Consider adding a daily smoothie to your diet as a way of increasing fruit and vegetable consumption, ensuring you include a leafy green vegetable, such as kale, as well as fruit.

4. Think about your favourite recipes and swap out meat for beans. This could be dishes like lentil bolognese, vegetable lasagna, tofu curry and bean chilli.

5. Add a tablespoon or two of ground flaxseeds (or linseeds) to your porridge, smoothie or soup, or sprinkle them on your salad.

6. Minimise processed foods and aim to cook from scratch as much as possible. This will not only be better for health but is usually cheaper. Bulk-buying dried staples and batch cooking can help too.

7. Swap refined grains with whole grains. This means changing from white bread to wholemeal bread, white rice to brown rice, white pasta to whole-wheat pasta. Include some lesser-known grains like buckwheat, teff, spelt, quinoa, millet and sorghum.

8. Drink mainly water for thirst. Drinking coffee and tea is also healthy if you enjoy it and are not overly sensitive to caffeine side-effects. Make green tea your tea of choice. Avoid sugar-sweetened beverages and even those with artificial sweeteners, as they can disrupt your gut bacteria. Minimise or avoid drinking alcohol.

9. If you snack during the day, make sure it's with fruit, vegetables, nuts and seeds. Aim to eat a 30 g portion of nuts on most days.

10. Focus daily on calcium-rich foods, including calcium-set tofu, low-oxalate leafy greens (such as arugula, romaine lettuce, mustard and collard greens, bok choy, kale, cabbage), beans, fortified plant milks and yoghurts.

11. Emphasise foods rich in iron, including chickpeas, lentils, tofu, cashew nuts, flaxseeds, pumpkin seeds, kale, dried apricots and raisins. Cooking with cast iron cookware can help increase intake. To increase absorption, eat iron-rich foods with a source of vitamin C. Avoid tea and coffee an hour before and after meals.

12. Don't eat too late in the evening or at night as this can adversely affect metabolic health.

13. Take a vitamin D3 tablet every day if you are not able to get enough exposure to the sun.

14. If you are following a 100% vegan or plant-based diet then make sure you are taking a B12 supplement and know where to get iodine in your diet (supplement, fortified foods or certain seaweeds).

15. Don't forget that many traditional cuisines, such as Indian, Mexican and African, are mostly plant-based already. Experiment with dishes from around the globe, incorporating plenty of herbs and spices.

Finally, find your 'tribe' and make sure you surround yourself with people who share your values, ethic and vision for a healthier future. It can be hard doing this alone and your chances of success will significantly increase with the right support. Always keep in mind your *Why*. Why is a transition to a plant-based diet important to you? This will keep you motivated and on the right path.

Abbreviations

AGE	advanced glycation end products
AHEI	Alternate Healthy Eating Index
AHS-2	Adventist Health Study-2
AIRC	American Institute for Cancer Research
ALA	alpha-linolenic acid
AMD	age-related macular degeneration
BCAA	branched chain amino acids
BMI	body mass index
BPA	bisphenol A
CA	Conservation Agriculture
CAC	coronary artery calcium
CAD	coronary artery disease
CARDIA	Coronary Artery Risk Development in Young People
CARDIVEG	Cardiovascular Prevention with Vegetarian Diet
CHD	coronary heart disease
CRP	C-reactive protein
CVD	cardiovascular disease
cyanCbl	cyanocobalamin
DART	Diet and Reinfarction Trial
DART-2	Diet and Angina Randomized Trial
DASH	Dietary Approaches to Stop Hypertension
DHA	docosahexaenoic acid

DIEFITS	Diet Intervention Examining the Factors Interacting with Treatment Success study
EPA	eicosapentaenoic acid
EPIC	European Prospective Investigation into Cancer and Nutrition
EVOO	extra-virgin olive oil
FAO	Food and Agriculture Organization
FMD	flow-mediated vasodilatation
FODMAPs	fermentable oligosaccharides, disaccharides, monosaccharides and polyols
FOS	Framingham Offspring Study
GHG	greenhouse gas
GEICO	Government Employees Insurance Company
HbA1c	haemoglobin A1C
HDL	high-density lipoprotein
HEALM	Hierarchies of Evidence Applied to Lifestyle Medicine
HELFIMED	Healthy Eating for Life with a Mediterranean Style Diet
holoTC	transcobalamin
HPFS	Health Professionals Follow-up Study
HRT	hormone replacement therapy
IARC	International Agency for Research on Cancer
IBS	irritable bowel syndrome
IGF-1	insulin-like growth factor
IPCC	Intergovernmental Panel on Climate Change
LDL	low-density lipoprotein
methylCbl	methylcobalamin
MUFA	monounsaturated fatty acid
NAFLD	non-alcoholic fatty liver disease
NHANES	National Health and Nutrition Examination Survey
NHS	National Health Service (UK)
PCOS	polycystic ovarian syndrome

Abbreviations

PBDI	plant-based diet index
PBMA	plant-based meat alternatives
PCBs	polychlorinated biphenyls
PCRM	Physician's Committee for Responsible Medicine
POP	persistent organic pollutants
PREDIMED	Prevention with Mediterranean Diet
PSA	prostate specific antigen
PUFA	polyunsaturated fatty acid
PURE	Prospective Urban Rural Epidemiology
RCT	randomised controlled trial
RDI	recommended daily intake
REDUCE-IT	Reduction of Cardiovascular Events with Icosapent Ethyl
ROS	reactive oxygen species
SCFA	short-chain fatty acids
SRI	system of rice intensification
TMA	trimethylamine
TMAO	trimethylamine oxide
TOFI	thin on the outside, fat on the inside
UTI	urinary tract infection
VeChi	Vegetarian and Vegan Children Study
WCRF	World Cancer Research Fund
WHO	World Health Organization
WFPB	whole food plant-based

Glossary

Advanced glycation end products: harmful compounds formed when cooking foods at high temperatures and also present in high amounts in animal foods such as red meat and poultry.

Alzheimer disease/dementia: the commonest form of dementia characterised by specific neuropathological abnormalities.

Amino acids: the building blocks of proteins. Organic compounds composed of nitrogen, carbon, hydrogen and oxygen, along with a variable side chain, which is specific to each amino acid.

Antioxidants: compounds that prevent damage from reactive oxygen species.

Atherosclerosis: a disease process by which plaque builds up in arteries. These plaques (**calcified atherosclerotic plaques**) are composed of fat, cholesterol and calcium. The plaque narrows the arteries and impairs blood flow to the organ being supplied by these arteries. This is the main cause of heart attacks and strokes.

Blue Zones: regions around the world where people live the longest, healthiest lives and are more likely to reach the age of 100 years. There are five Blue Zones: Loma Linda

Eating Plant-Based

in California, Ikaria in Greece, Sardinia in Italy, Nicoya Peninsula in Costa Rica and Okinawa in Japan.

Branched chain amino acids: leucine isoleucine and valine.

Calcified atherosclerotic plaques: calcium-containing, fatty plaques in the arteries.

Carcinogen: a substance capable of causing cancer.

Cardio-metabolic diseases: a group of common and often preventable diseases including heart disease, stroke, type 2 diabetes, insulin resistance and non-alcoholic fatty liver.

Cardiovascular disease (CVD): a general term referring to conditions affecting the heart and blood vessels. It most commonly refers to heart disease (myocardial infarction, heart failure), hypertension and stroke.

Carotenoids: yellow, orange and red pigments synthesised by plants, including alpha-carotene, beta-carotene, beta-cryptoxanthin, lutein, zeaxanthin and lycopene. These compounds have antioxidant properties.

Cholesterol: a fat-life substance present in the blood. The structure is really a modified steroid attached to an alcohol. Cholesterol is an essential part of animal cell membranes and is required for synthesis of bile acids, steroid hormones (oestrogen, testosterone and hormones made by the adrenal gland) and vitamin D. The liver can make all the cholesterol that the body requires. It is not required in the diet. It is carried through the blood attached to proteins. This combination of proteins and cholesterol is called a lipoprotein. There are different types of cholesterol based on what the lipoprotein carries. On a very basic level this includes **low-density lipoprotein (LDL)** cholesterol, which transports cholesterol particles throughout the body, and **high-density lipoprotein (HDL)**, which picks up excess cholesterol and takes it back to the liver.

Coronary arteries: the arteries supplying the heart.

Cruciferous vegetables: of the *Brassicaceae* family and whose flowers are shaped like a cross.

Dementia: a general term used to describe a decline in mental and cognitive ability.

Eco-Atkins: plant-based low-carbohydrate diet.

Essential amino acids: nine amino acids that cannot be made by the human body and have to be obtained from the diet. These are histidine, isoleucine, leucine, lysine, methionine, phenylalanine, threonine, tryptophan and valine.

Flavonoids: a large family of polyphenolic compounds found in plants giving them their vibrant colours and which have antioxidant properties.

Flow-mediated dilatation: widening of an artery when blood flows increases.

HDL-cholesterol: (high-density lipoprotein cholesterol) is considered to be a 'good' type of cholesterol. Higher levels are considered beneficial.

High-oxalate greens: spinach, Swiss chard, beet greens, rhubarb leaves.

Hyperlipidaemia/dyslipidaemia: abnormally high blood lipid (fat) levels, including high cholesterol and high triglycerides.

Hypertension: persistent elevation in blood pressure. Ideal blood pressure is considered to be 90/60 mm Hg to 120/80 mm Hg. The traditional definition of hypertension has been a blood pressure of 140/90 mm Hg or higher, but these criteria are being lowered with any blood pressure over 120/80 mm Hg considered unhealthy.

Iliac arteries: provide the blood supply to the legs, reproductive system and pelvic region.

Insulin resistance: when cells in your body are unable to respond to insulin and therefore cannot take up glucose. This is the main cause of type 2 diabetes but occurs in a number of related conditions.

Ischaemic/ischaemia: is a restriction in the blood supply to tissues causing a lack of oxygen. Ischaemia is generally caused by problems with the blood vessels, such as blockage by atherosclerotic plaques, with resulting damage to or death of the tissue.

Ischaemic heart disease/coronary heart disease/coronary artery disease: interchangeable terms for a condition where the blood vessels supplying the heart (coronary arteries) are narrowed or blocked due to the development of atherosclerosis. This can lead to angina and heart attacks.

Isoflavones: flavonoids that have oestrogen-like properties and are also referred to as phyto-oestrogens (plant oestrogens).

LDL-cholesterol: (low-density lipoprotein cholesterol) considered an unhealthy form of cholesterol. It is a direct cause of atherosclerosis and higher levels are associated with an increased risk of heart attack and stroke.

Linseed: same as flaxseed.

Meta-analysis: an analysis that combines the results of a number of research studies.

Metabolic syndrome: refers to having a number of risk factors that put you at risk of type 2 diabetes and cardiovascular disease. The definition varies but one definition involves having three of the following five criteria: abdominal obesity, high blood triglyceride levels, low HDL-cholesterol, high blood pressure and high fasting glucose.

Microbiome: the trillions of microorganisms that line our body.

Glossary

Myocardial infarction: known as a heart attack. Usually occurs when an atherosclerotic plaque in a coronary artery ruptures and the resulting blood clot that forms decreases or stops the blood flow to a part of the heart causing damage or death of that part of the heart muscle.

Nitric oxide: a compound made by the body that results in vasodilation – widening of the blood vessels.

Oligosaccharides: a group of a few sugar molecules, usually between three and 10 simple sugars or 'monosaccharides'.

Oxalates: or oxalic compounds in food can inhibit the absorption of nutrients such as calcium.

Phytates or phytic acid is the main store of phosphate in plants.

Phytonutrients: naturally occurring nutrients found in plants.

Phyto-oestrogens: plant oestrogens, including isoflavones and lignans.

Plant-based or plant-based diet: a general term referring to diet patterns that are predominantly based around whole plant foods. In this book it includes a whole food plant-based diet, vegetarian and vegan diet patterns.

Polyphenols: compounds naturally found in plants that have antioxidant and anti-inflammatory properties.

Prebiotics: substances that induce the growth or action of our gut microbiota.

Probiotics: live microorganisms that confer health benefits on human when administered in adequate amounts.

Pseudograins: have the appearance of grains but botanically they are not grains but from a different plant family (not a grass). Nonetheless, they are still often referred to as grains. This includes amaranth, buckwheat, quinoa, wild rice and kaniwa.

Ruminant animals: a group of herbivorous animals that have a stomach with four compartments and are consequently able to digest plant foods, such as grass, through fermentation by bacteria in their stomach. This process of digestion produces methane, a greenhouse gas.

Sarcopenia: degenerative loss of skeletal muscle mass, quality and strength associated with age.

Soil meso-fauna: invertebrate animals that live in the soil and feed on a variety of plants, animals and insects found in the soil, supporting its overall health.

Stroke: a life-threatening medical condition in which the blood supply to a part of the brain is cut off.

Tocopherols: a group of compounds with vitamin E-like properties.

Triglycerides: a type of fat in the blood. When excess calories are consumed they are converted to triglycerides which are stored in your fat cells but can also be stored inside liver and muscle cells, causing insulin resistance.

Type 2 diabetes: a chronic disease resulting in high blood glucose levels due to the body being unable to use the insulin it has produced effectively **(insulin resistance)** or being unable to produce enough insulin.

Vegan: an ethical choice not to eat or use any animal products.

Vegetarian: a diet pattern that excludes all meat and fish but still includes eggs and dairy.

Whole food plant-based diet: consists of minimally processed fruit, vegetables, whole grains, legumes, nuts and seeds, herbs and spices and excludes all (or most) animal products, including red meat, poultry, fish, eggs and dairy products.

Zoonoses: infections that have jumped from a non-human species to humans.

Resources

Plant-Based Health Professionals UK (PBHP UK)

PBHP UK was founded in 2018 by Dr Shireen Kassam. It is a community interest company, based in the UK, and is increasingly receiving international recognition. PBHP UK's mission is to provide education and advocacy on whole food plant-based nutrition for the prevention and treatment of chronic disease. This education is inclusive of health professionals, general public and policy makers. PBHP UK is a membership organisation open to everyone, not just health professionals, and aims to develop a strong network of likeminded individuals who are empowered to spread the plant-based message. On the website you can find numerous free resources including factsheets, articles, videos, recipes and a 21-day plant-based health challenge.

The PBHP UK team launched the UK's first regulated plant-based lifestyle medicine service in January 2021, Plant Based Health Online. This service provides one-to-one and group consultations for patients and clients who are looking to regain their health and thrive using a plant-based lifestyle approach. It is available throughout the UK and beyond.

https://plantbasedhealthprofessionals.com
https://plantbasedhealthonline.com

Plant-Based Canada

Plant-Based Canada is a non-profit organisation co-founded by Dr Zahra Kassam and Michelle Fedele RD in 2019. Our mission and guiding principles are to provide education to the public, health professionals and policy makers, on the evidence-based benefits of whole food plant-based nutrition that is sustainable and the healthiest possible, which also promotes the well-being of the planet and all its lifeforms, and to collaborate with sister organisations with the same mission.

www.plantbasedcanada.org

All proceeds from the book will be divided between these two organisations and used directly to continue their work.

References

Chapter 1: Eating plant-based

1.   GBD Diet Collaborators. Health effects of dietary risks in 195 countries, 1990–2017: a systematic analysis for the Global Burden of Disease Study 2017. *Lancet* 2019; 393(10184): P1958-P1972. doi.org/10.1016/S0140-6736(19)30041-8

2.   Poore J, Nemecek T. Reducing food's environmental impacts through producers and consumers. *Science* 2018; 360(6392): 987-992. doi:10.1126/science.aaq0216

3.   Dinu M, Abbate R, Gensini GF, Casini A, Sofi F. Vegetarian, vegan diets and multiple health outcomes: A systematic review with meta-analysis of observational studies. *Crit Rev Food Sci Nutr* 2017; 57(17): 3640-3649. doi:10.1080/10408398.2016.1138447

4.   Tong TYN, Appleby PN, Bradbury KE, et al. Risks of ischaemic heart disease and stroke in meat eaters, fish eaters, and vegetarians over 18 years of follow-up: Results from the prospective EPIC-Oxford study. *Br Med J* 2019; 366: 14897. doi:10.1136/bmj.l4897

5.   Satija A, Bhupathiraju SN, Spiegelman D, et al. Healthful and Unhealthful Plant-Based Diets and the Risk of Coronary Heart Disease in U.S. Adults. *J Am Coll Cardiol* 2017; 70(4): 411-422. doi:10.1016/j.jacc.2017.05.047

6.   Papier K, Appleby PN, Fensom G, Knuppel A, et al. Vegetarian diets and risk of hospitalisation or death with diabetes in British adults: results from the EPIC-Oxford study. *Nutr Diabetes* 2019; 9(1): 7. doi: 10.1038/s41387-019-0074-0

7.   Tonstad S, Butler T, Yan R, Fraser GE. Type of vegetarian diet, body weight, and prevalence of type 2 diabetes. *Diabetes Care* 2009; 32(5): 791-796. doi:10.2337/dc08-1886

8.   Satija A, Bhupathiraju SN, Rimm ER, et al. Plant-Based Dietary Patterns and Incidence of Type 2 Diabetes in US Men and Women: Results from Three Prospective Cohort Studies. *PLoS Med* 2016; 13(6): e1002039.

doi:10.1371/journal.pmed.1002039

9. Appleby PN, Davey GK, Key TJ. Hypertension and blood pressure among meat eaters, fish eaters, vegetarians and vegans in EPIC–Oxford. *Public Health Nutr* 2002; 5(5): 645-654. doi:10.1079/phn2002332

10. Bradbury KE, Crowe FL, Appleby PN, et al. Serum concentrations of cholesterol, apolipoprotein A-I and apolipoprotein B in a total of 1694 meat-eaters, fish-eaters, vegetarians and vegans. *Eur J Clin Nutr* 2014; 68: 178-183. doi:10.1038/ejcn.2013.248

11. Yokoyama Y, Nishimura K, Barnard ND. Vegetarian diets and blood pressure ameta-analysis. *JAMA Intern Med* 2014; 174(4): 577-587. doi:10.1001/jamainternmed.2013.14547

12. Jenkins DJA, Jones PJH, Lamarche B. Effect of a dietary portfolio of cholesterol-lowering foods given at 2 levels of intensity of dietary advice on serum lipids in hyperlipidemia: A randomized controlled trial. *JAMA* 2011; 306(8): 831-839. doi:10.1001/jama.2011.1202

13. Chiavaroli L, Nishi SK, Khan TA, et al. Portfolio Dietary Pattern and Cardiovascular Disease: A Systematic Review and Meta-analysis of Controlled Trials. *Progress in Cardiovascular Diseases* 2018; 61(1): 43-53. doi:10.1016/j.pcad.2018.05.004

14. Barnard ND, Cohen J, Jenkins DJA, et al. A low-fat vegan diet and a conventional diabetes diet in the treatment of type 2 diabetes: A randomized, controlled, 74-wk clinical trial. *Am J Clin Nutr* 2009; 89(5): 1588S-1596S. doi:10.3945/ajcn.2009.26736H

15. Garber AJ, Handelsman Y, Grunberger G, et al. Consensus statement by the American Association of clinical Endocrinologists and American College of Endocrinology on the comprehensive type 2 diabetes management algorithm - 2020 executive summary. *Endocrine Practice* 2020; 26(1): 107-139. doi:10.4158/CS-2019-0472

16. Kelly J, Karlsen M, Steinke G. Type 2 Diabetes Remission and Lifestyle Medicine: A Position Statement From the American College of Lifestyle Medicine. *Am J Lifestyle Med* 2020; 14(4): 406-419. doi: 10.1177/1559827620930962.

17. Ornish D, Scherwitz LW, Billings JH, et al. Intensive lifestyle changes for reversal of coronary heart disease. *J Am Med Assoc* 1998; 280(23): 2001-2007. doi:10.1001/jama.280.23.2001

18. Esselstyn CB, Gendy G, Doyle J, Golubic M, Roizen MF. A way to reverse CAD? *J Fam Pract* 2014; 63(7): 356-364b. PMID: 25198208.

19. Gupta SK, Sawhney RC, Rai L, et al. Regression of Coronary Atherosclerosis through Healthy Lifestyle in Coronary Artery Disease Patients - Mount Abu Open Heart Trial. *Indian Heart J* 2011; 63(5): 461–469.

20. Frattaroli J, Weider G, Dnistrian AM, et al. Clinical Events in Prostate Cancer Lifestyle Trial: Results From Two Years of Follow-Up. *Urology* 2008; 72(6): 1319-1323. doi:10.1016/j.urology.2008.04.050

21. Katz ET. Dr. Dean Ornish Explains The Reason For Bill Clinton's Diet

References

Change. *HuffPost* 24 April 2014.
www.huffpost.com/entry/bill-clinton-diet_n_5208245

22. Database, M. coverage. Decision Memo for Intensive Cardiac Rehabilitation (ICR) Program - Dr. Ornish's Program for Reversing Heart Disease (CAG-00419N). 14 May 2010.
www.cms.gov/medicare-coverage-database/view/nca.aspx

23. Orlich MJ, et al. Vegetarian Epidemiology: Review and Discussion of Findings from Geographically Diverse Cohorts. *Adv Nutr* 2019. doi:10.1093/advances/nmy109

24. Satija A, Bhupathiraju SN, Spiegelman D, et al. Healthful and Unhealthful Plant-Based Diets and the Risk of Coronary Heart Disease in U.S. Adults. *J Am Coll Cardiol* 2017; 70(4): 411-422. doi:10.1016/j.jacc.2017.05.047

25. Kane-Diallo A, Srour B, Sellem L, et al. Association between a pro plant-based dietary score and cancer risk in the prospective NutriNet-santé cohort. *Int J Cancer* 2018; 143(9): 2168-2176. doi:10.1002/ijc.31593

26. Mazidi M, Kengne AP. Higher adherence to plant-based diets are associated with lower likelihood of fatty liver. *Clin Nutr* 2019; 38(4): 1672-1677. doi: 10.1016/j.clnu.2018.08.010

27. Satija A, Bhupathiraju SN, Rimm EB, et al. Plant-Based Dietary Patterns and Incidence of Type 2 Diabetes in US Men and Women: Results from Three Prospective Cohort Studies. *PLoS Med* 2016; 13(6): e1002039. doi:10.1371/journal.pmed.1002039

28. Kim H, Caulfield LE, Garcia-Larsen V, et al. Plant-based diets and incident CKD and kidney function. *Clin J Am Soc Nephrol* 2019; 14(5): 682-691. doi:10.2215/CJN.12391018

29. Jafari S, Hezaveh E, Jalilpiran Y, et al. Plant-based diets and risk of disease mortality: a systematic review and meta-analysis of cohort studies. *Crit Rev Food Sci Nutr* 2021 May 6; 1-13. doi:10.1080/10408398.2021.1918628

30. Satija A, Yu E, Willett WC, Hu FB. Understanding Nutritional Epidemiology and Its Role in Policy. *Adv Nutr* 2015; 6(1): 5-18. doi:10.3945/an.114.007492

31. Dinu M, Abbate R, Gensini GF, Casini A, Sofi F. Vegetarian, vegan diets and multiple health outcomes: A systematic review with meta-analysis of observational studies. *Crit Rev Food Sci Nutr* 2017; 57(17) 3640-3649. doi:10.1080/10408398.2016.1138447

32. Allen NE, Appleby PN, Davey GK, et al. The associations of diet with serum insulin-like growth factor I and its main binding proteins in 292 women meat-eaters, vegetarians, and vegans. *Cancer Epidemiol Biomarkers Prev* 2002; 11(11): 1441-1448. PMID: 12433724.

33. Askie L, Offringa M. Systematic reviews and meta-analysis. *Semin Fetal Neonatal Med* 2015; 20(6): 403-409. doi:10.1016/j.siny.2015.10.002

34. Vesper I. Mass resignation guts board of prestigious Cochrane Collaboration. *Nature* 17 September 2018. doi:10.1038/d41586-018-06727-0

35. Katz D, Karlsen M, Chung M, et al. Hierarchies of Evidence Applied to

Lifestyle Medicine (HEALM): Introduction of a Strength-of-evidence Approach Based on a Methodological Systematic Review (P13-023-19). *Curr Dev Nutr* 2019; 3(Suppl 1): 13-23. doi: 10.1093/cdn/nzz036.P13-023-19

36. Katz DL, Karlsen MC, Chung M, et al. Hierarchies of evidence applied to lifestyle Medicine (HEALM): Introduction of a strength-of-evidence approach based on a methodological systematic review. *BMC Medical Research Methodology* 2019; 19: 178. doi.org/10.1186/s12874-019-0811-z

37. Anglemyer A, Horvath HT, Bero L. Healthcare outcomes assessed with observational study designs compared with those assessed in randomized trials. *Cochrane Database Syst Rev* 2014; 2014(4): MR000034. doi: 10.1002/14651858.MR000034.pub2.

38. Konner M, Boyd Eaton S. Paleolithic nutrition: Twenty-five years later. *Nutr Clin Pract* 2010; 25(6): 594-602. doi:10.1177/0884533610385702

39. Storhaug CL, Fosse SK, Fadnes LT. Country, regional, and global estimates for lactose malabsorption in adults: a systematic review and meta-analysis. *Lancet Gastroenterol Hepatol* 2017; 2(10): 738-746. doi:10.1016/S2468-1253(17)30154-1

40. Itan Y, Powell A, Beaumont MA, Burger J, Thomas MG. The origins of lactase persistence in Europe. *PLoS Comput Biol* 2009; 5(8): e1000491. doi:10.1371/journal.pcbi.1000491

41. Buettner D, Skemp S. Blue Zones: Lessons From the World's Longest Lived. *Am J Lifestyle Med* 2016; 10(5): 318-321. doi:10.1177/1559827616637066

42. Crowley J, Ball L, Hiddink GJ. Nutrition in medical education: a systematic review. *Lancet Planet Heal* 2019; 3(9): e379-e389. doi:10.1016/S2542-5196(19)30171-8

43. Devries S, Willett W, Bonow RO. Nutrition Education in Medical School, Residency Training, and Practice. *JAMA* 2019; 321(14): 1351-1352. doi:10.1001/jama.2019.1581

44. Sauerteig SO, Wijesuriya J, Tuck M, Barham-Brown H. Doctors' health and wellbeing: at the heart of the NHS's mission or still a secondary consideration? *Int Rev Psychiatry* 2019; 31(7-8): 548-554. doi:10.1080/09540261.2019.1586165

45. Lobelo F, Duperly J, Frank E. Physical activity habits of doctors and medical students influence their counselling practices. *Br J Sports Med* 2009; 43(2): 89-92. doi:10.1136/bjsm.2008.055426

46. Macaninch E, Buckner L, Amin P, et al. Time for nutrition in medical education. *BMJ Nutr Prev Health* 2020; 3: e000049. doi:bmjnph-2019-000049. doi: 10.1136/bmjnph-2019-000049

47. Hark LA, Deen D. Position of the Academy of Nutrition and Dietetics: Interprofessional Education in Nutrition as an Essential Component of Medical Education. *J Acad Nutr Diet* 2017; 117(7): 1104-1113. doi:10.1016/j.jand.2017.04.019

48. Lenfant C. Clinical Research to Clinical Practice — Lost in Translation? *N*

References

Engl J Med 2003; 349: 868-874. doi:10.1056/nejmsa035507

49. Willett W, Rockstrom J, Loken B, et al. Food in the Anthropocene: the EAT–Lancet Commission on healthy diets from sustainable food systems. *Lancet* 2019; 393(10170): 447-492. doi.org/10.1016/S0140-6736(18)31788-4

50. Melina V, Craig W, Levin S. Position of the Academy of Nutrition and Dietetics: Vegetarian Diets. *J Acad Nutr Diet* 2016; 116(2): 1970-1980. doi:10.1016/j.jand.2016.09.025

51. Swinburn BA, Kraak VI, Allender S, et al. The Global Syndemic of Obesity, Undernutrition, and Climate Change: The Lancet Commission report. *Lancet* 2019; 393(10173): 791-846. doi.org/10.1016/S0140-6736(18)32822-8

52. Hall KD, Guo J, Courville AB, et al. Effect of a plant-based, low-fat diet versus an animal-based, ketogenic diet on ad libitum energy intake. *Nat Med* 2021; 27(2): 344-353. doi:10.1038/s41591-020-01209-1

53. Barnard ND, Alwarith J, Rembert E, et al. A Mediterranean Diet and Low-Fat Vegan Diet to Improve Body Weight and Cardiometabolic Risk Factors: A Randomized, Cross-over Trial. *J Am Coll Nutr* 2021; 1-13. doi:10.1080/07315724.2020.1869625

54. Kahleova H, Petersen KF, Shulman GI, Shulman GI. Effect of a Low-Fat Vegan Diet on Body Weight, Insulin Sensitivity, Postprandial Metabolism, and Intramyocellular and Hepatocellular Lipid Levels in Overweight Adults. *JAMA Netw Open* 2020; 3.

55. Kahleova H, Petersen KF, Shulman GI, et al. Effect of a Low-Fat Vegan Diet on Body Weight, Insulin Sensitivity, Postprandial Metabolism, and Intramyocellular and Hepatocellular Lipid Levels in Overweight Adults: A Randomized Clinical Trial. *JAMA Netw Open* 2020; 3(11): e2025454. doi:10.1001/jamanetworkopen.2020.25454

56. Klementova M, Thieme L, Haluzik M, et al. A plant-based meal increases gastrointestinal hormones and satiety more than an energy-and macronutrient-matched processed-meat meal in t2d, obese, and healthy men: A three-group randomized crossover study. *Nutrients* 2019; 11(1): 157. doi: 10.3390/nu11010157

57. Kahleova H, Tura A, Klementova M, et al. A plant-based meal stimulates incretin and insulin secretion more than an energy-and macronutrient-matched standard meal in type 2 diabetes: A randomized crossover study. *Nutrients* 2019; 11(3): 486. doi:10.3390/nu11030486

58. Huang RY, Huang CC, Hu FB, Chavarro JE. Vegetarian Diets and Weight Reduction: a Meta-Analysis of Randomized Controlled Trials. *J Gen Intern Med* 2016; 31(1): 109-116. doi:10.1007/s11606-015-3390-7

59. Vergnaud A-C, Norat T, Romaguera D, et al. Meat consumption and prospective weight change in participants of the EPIC-PANACEA study. *Am J Clin Nutr* 2010; 92(2): 398-407. doi:10.3945/ajcn.2009.28713

60. Satija A, Malik V, Rimm EB, et al. Changes in intake of plant-based diets and weight change: Results from 3 prospective cohort studies. *Am J Clin Nutr* 2019; 110(3): 574-582. doi:10.1093/ajcn/nqz049

61. Barnard ND, Levin SM, Yokoyama Y. A Systematic Review and Meta-Analysis of Changes in Body Weight in Clinical Trials of Vegetarian Diets. *J Acad Nutr Diet* 2015; 115(6): 954-969. doi:10.1016/j.jand.2014.11.016

62. Wright N, Wilson L, Smith M, Duncan B, McHugh P. The BROAD study: A randomised controlled trial using a whole food plant-based diet in the community for obesity, ischaemic heart disease or diabetes. *Nutr Diabetes* 2017; 7(3): e256. doi:10.1038/nutd.2017.3

63. Tomova A, Bukovsky I, Rembert E, et al. The Effects of Vegetarian and Vegan Diets on Gut Microbiota . *Frontiers in Nutrition* 2019; 6, 47. doi.org/10.3389/fnut.2019.00047

64. Trichopoulou A, Bamia C, Trichopoulos D. Anatomy of health effects of Mediterranean diet: Greek EPIC prospective cohort study. *Br Med J* 2009; 338. doi:10.1136/bmj.b2337

65. Estruch R, Ros E, Salas-Salvado J, et al. Primary Prevention of Cardiovascular Disease with a Mediterranean Diet Supplemented with Extra-Virgin Olive Oil or Nuts. *N Engl J Med* 2018; 378: e34. doi:10.1056/NEJMoa1800389

66. Martínez-González MA, Sanchez-Tainta A, Corella D, et al. A provegetarian food pattern and reduction in total mortality in the Prevención con Dieta Mediterránea (PREDIMED) study. *Am J Clin Nutr* 2014; 100(Suppl 1): 320S-3208S. doi:10.3945/ajcn.113.071431

67. Pagliai G, Dinu M, Mangino A, et al. Comparison between Mediterranean and Vegetarian diets for cardiovascular prevention: The cardiveg study. *Cochrane Library: Nutr Metab Cardiovasc Dis* 2017; 2017(4). doi:10.1016/j.numecd.2016.11.084

68. Sofi F, Dinu M, Pagliai G, et al. Low-calorie vegetarian versus mediterranean diets for reducing body weight and improving cardiovascular risk profile. *Circulation* 2018; 137(11): 1103-1113. doi:10.1161/CIRCULATIONAHA.117.030088

69. Rogerson D, Maçãs D, Milner M, Liu Y, Klonizakis M. Contrasting effects of short-term mediterranean and vegan diets on microvascular function and cholesterol in younger adults: A comparative pilot study. *Nutrients* 2018; 10(2): 1897. doi:10.3390/nu10121897

70. Ornish D, Brown SE, Scherwitz LW, et al. Can lifestyle changes reverse coronary heart disease?. The Lifestyle Heart Trial. *Lancet* 1990; 336(8708): 129-133. doi:10.1016/0140-6736(90)91656-U

71. Tsaban G, Meir AY, Rinott E, et al. The effect of green Mediterranean diet on cardiometabolic risk; A randomised controlled trial. *Heart* 2020 Nov 23. doi:10.1136/heartjnl-2020-317802

72. Yaskolka Meir A, Rinott E, Tsaban G, et al. Effect of green-Mediterranean diet on intrahepatic fat: the DIRECT PLUS randomised controlled trial. *Gut* 2021; 70(11): 2085-2095. doi:10.1136/gutjnl-2020-323106

73. Willcox DC, Scapagnini G, Willcox BJ. Healthy aging diets other than the Mediterranean: A focus on the Okinawan diet. *Mech Ageing Dev* 2014; 136-137: 148-162. doi:10.1016/j.mad.2014.01.002

References

74. Jenkins DJA, Wong JMW, Kendall CWC, et al. Effect of a 6-month vegan low-carbohydrate ('Eco-Atkins') diet on cardiovascular risk factors and body weight in hyperlipidaemic adults: A randomised controlled trial. *BMJ Open* 2014; 4: e003505. doi:10.1136/bmjopen-2013-003505

75. Seidelmann SB, Claggett B, Cheng A, et al. Dietary carbohydrate intake and mortality: a prospective cohort study and meta-analysis. *Lancet Public Heal* 2018; 3(9): E419-E428. doi:10.1016/S2468-2667(18)30135-X

76. Mazidi M, Katsiki N, Mikhailidis DP, Sattar N, Banach M. Lower carbohydrate diets and all-cause and cause-specific mortality: A population-based cohort study and pooling of prospective studies. *Eur Heart J* 2019; 40(34): 2870-2879. doi:10.1093/eurheartj/ehz174

77. Hall KD, Chen KY, Guo J, et al. Energy expenditure and body composition changes after an isocaloric ketogenic diet in overweight and obese men. *Am J Clin Nutr* 2016; 104(2): 324-333. doi:10.3945/ajcn.116.133561

78. Holt SHA, Miller JC, Petocz P. An insulin index of foods: The insulin demand generated by 1000-kJ portions of common foods. *Am J Clin Nutr* 1997; 66(5): 1264-1276. doi:10.1093/ajcn/66.5.1264

79. Hannou SA, Haslam DE, McKeown NM, Herman MA. Fructose metabolism and metabolic disease. *J Clin Investig* 2018; 128(2): 545-555. doi: 10.1172/JCI96702

80. Mai BH, Yan L-J. The negative and detrimental effects of high fructose on the liver, with special reference to metabolic disorders. *Diabetes Metab Syndr Obes* 2019; 12: 821-826. doi:10.2147/DMSO.S198968

81. Lowette K, Roosen L, Tack J, Vanden Berghe P. Effects of High-Fructose Diets on Central Appetite Signaling and Cognitive Function. *Frontiers in Nutrition* 2015; 2: 5. doi:10.3389/fnut.2015.00005

82. Lustig RH. Fructose: It's 'alcohol without the buzz'. *Adv Nutr* 2013; 4(2): 226-235. doi:10.3945/an.112.002998

83. Kearns CE, Schmidt LA, Glantz SA. Sugar industry and coronary heart disease research: A historical analysis of internal industry documents. *JAMA Intern Med* 2016; 176(11): 1680-1685. doi:10.1001/jamainternmed.2016.5394

84. Rauber F, Da Costa ML, Steele EM, et al. Ultra-processed food consumption and chronic non-communicable diseases-related dietary nutrient profile in the UK (2008–2014). *Nutrients* 2018; 10(5): 587. doi:10.3390/nu10050587

85. Nardocci M, Leclerc B-S, Louzada M-L, et al. Consumption of ultra-processed foods and obesity in Canada. *Can J Public Health* 2019; 110(1): 4-14. doi:10.17269/s41997-018-0130-x

86. Scarborough P, Kaur A, Cobiac L, et al. Eatwell Guide: Modelling the dietary and cost implications of incorporating new sugar and fibre guidelines. *BMJ Open* 2016; 6(12): e013182. doi:10.1136/bmjopen-2016-013182

87. Bernstein AM, Bloom DE, Rosner BA, Franz M, Willett WC. Relation of

food cost to healthfulness of diet among US women. *Am J Clin Nutr* 2010; 92(5): 1197-1203. doi:10.3945/ajcn.2010.29854

88. Flynn MM, Schiff AR. Economical Healthy Diets (2012): Including Lean Animal Protein Costs More Than Using Extra Virgin Olive Oil. *J Hunger Environ Nutr* 2015; 10(4): 467-482. doi:10.1080/19320248.2015.1045675

89. The Food Foundation. *The Broken Plate 2021;The State of the Nations Food System*. 6 July 2021.
https://foodfoundation.org.uk/publication/broken-plate-2021

90. Canada's Food Price Report 11th Edition 2021. (2021).
https://niagaraknowledgeexchange.com/wp-content/uploads/sites/2/2021/01/Canada-Food-Price-Report-2021-EN-December-8.pdf

91. Lin CL, Wang JH, Lin MN, Chang CC, Chiu THT. Vegetarian diets and medical expenditure in taiwan—a matched cohort study. *Nutrients* 2019; 11(11): 2688. doi:10.3390/nu11112688

92. Arnett DK, Blumenthal RS, Albert MA, et al. 2019 ACC/AHA Guideline on the Primary Prevention of Cardiovascular Disease: A Report of the American College of Cardiology/American Heart Association Task Force on Clinical Practice Guidelines. *Circulation* 2019; 140(11): e596-e646. doi:10.1161/CIR.0000000000000678

93. Evert AB, Dennison M, Gardner CD, et al. Nutrition therapy for adults with diabetes or prediabetes: A consensus report. *Diabetes Care* 2019; 42(5): 731-754. doi:10.2337/dci19-0014

94. Rock CL, Thomson C, Gansler T, et al. American Cancer Society guideline for diet and physical activity for cancer prevention. *CA Cancer J Clin* 2020; 70(4): 245-271. doi:10.3322/caac.21591

95. NHS Choices. The Eatwell Guide - Live Well - NHS Choices. UK (2016). doi:10.1016/j.talanta.2006.05.076

96. Health Canada. Canada's Dietary Guidelines. 22 January 2019.
https://food-guide.canada.ca/en/guidelines/

Chapter 2: Eating meat

1. Katz DL, Doughty KN, Geagan K, Jenkins DA, Gardner CD. Perspective: The Public Health Case for Modernizing the Definition of Protein Quality. *Advances in Nutrition* 2019. doi:10.1093/advances/nmz023

2. Miousse IR, et al. Modulation of dietary methionine intake elicits potent, yet distinct, anticancer effects on primary versus metastatic tumors. *Carcinogenesis* 2018. doi:10.1093/carcin/bgy085

3. Flores-Guerrero J, et al. Plasma Branched-Chain Amino Acids and Risk of Incident Type 2 Diabetes: Results from the PREVEND Prospective Cohort Study. *J Clin Med* 2018. doi:10.3390/jcm7120513

4. Rebholz CM, et al. Dietary Acid Load and Incident Chronic Kidney Disease: Results from the ARIC Study. *Am J Nephrol* 2015. doi:10.1159/000443746

5. Young VR. Soy protein in relation to human protein and amino acid nutrition. *J Am Dietetic Assoc* 1991.

6. Song M, et al. Association of animal and plant protein intake with all-cause and cause-specific mortality. *JAMA Intern Med* 2016. doi:10.1001/jamainternmed.2016.4182

7. Qi XX, Shen P. Associations of dietary protein intake with all-cause, cardiovascular disease, and cancer mortality: A systematic review and meta-analysis of cohort studies. *Nutr Metab Cardiovasc Dis* 2020. doi:10.1016/j.numecd.2020.03.008

8. Budhathoki S, et al. Association of Animal and Plant Protein Intake with All-Cause and Cause-Specific Mortality in a Japanese Cohort. *JAMA Intern Med* 2019. doi:10.1001/jamainternmed.2019.2806

9. Huang J, et al. Association between Plant and Animal Protein Intake and Overall and Cause-Specific Mortality. *JAMA Intern Med* 2020. doi:10.1001/jamainternmed.2020.2790

10. Zhong VW, et al. Associations of Processed Meat, Unprocessed Red Meat, Poultry, or Fish Intake with Incident Cardiovascular Disease and All-Cause Mortality. *JAMA Intern Med* 2020. doi:10.1001/jamainternmed.2019.6969

11. Naghshi S, Sadeghi O, Willett WC, Esmaillzadeh A. Dietary intake of total, animal, and plant proteins and risk of all cause, cardiovascular, and cancer mortality: Systematic review and dose-response meta-analysis of prospective cohort studies. *Br Med J* 2020. doi:10.1136/bmj.m2412

12. Zhong VW, et al. Protein foods from animal sources, incident cardiovascular disease and all-cause mortality: A substitution analysis. *Int J Epidemiol* 2021; 50.

13. Buitrago-Lopez A, et al. Chocolate consumption and cardiometabolic disorders: Systematic review and meta-analysis. *Br Med J* 2011. doi:10.1136/bmj.d4488

14. Sacks FM, et al. Dietary fats and cardiovascular disease: A presidential advisory from the American Heart Association. *Circulation* 2017. doi:10.1161/CIR.0000000000000510

15. Keys A, et al. The diet and 15-year death rate in the seven countries study. *Am J Epidemiol* 1986. doi:10.1093/oxfordjournals.aje.a114480

16. Siri-Tarino PW, Sun Q, Hu FB, Krauss RM. Meta-analysis of prospective cohort studies evaluating the association of saturated fat with cardiovascular disease. *Am J Clin Nutr* 2010. doi:10.3945/ajcn.2009.27725

17. Chowdhury R, et al. Association of dietary, circulating, and supplement fatty acids with coronary risk: A systematic review and meta-analysis. *Ann Intern Med* 2014. doi:10.7326/M13-1788

18. Ludwig DS, Willett WC, Volek JS, Neuhouser ML. Dietary fat: From foe to friend? *Science* 2018. doi:10.1126/science.aau2096

19. Dehghan M, et al. Associations of fats and carbohydrate intake with cardiovascular disease and mortality in 18 countries from five continents (PURE): a prospective cohort study. *Lancet* 2017; 390.

20. Dehghan M, et al. Association of dairy intake with cardiovascular disease and mortality in 21 countries from five continents (PURE): a prospective cohort study. *Lancet* 2018; 392.

21. Miller, V. et al. Fruit, vegetable, and legume intake, and cardiovascular disease and deaths in 18 countries (PURE): a prospective cohort study. *Lancet* 2017; 390:.

22. Han MA, et al. Reduction of red and processed meat intake and cancer mortality and incidence a systematic review and meta-analysis of cohort studies. *Ann Intern Med* 2019. doi:10.7326/M19-0699

23. Vernooij RWM, et al. Patterns of red and processed meat consumption and risk for cardiometabolic and cancer outcomes a systematic review and meta-analysis of cohort studies. *Ann Intern Med* 2019. doi:10.7326/M19-1583

24. Astrup A, et al. Saturated Fats and Health: A Reassessment and Proposal for Food-Based Recommendations: JACC State-of-the-Art Review. *J Am Coll Cardiology* 2020. doi:10.1016/j.jacc.2020.05.077

25. Valli C, et al. Health-related values and preferences regarding meat consumption a mixed-methods systematic review. *Annals of Internal Medicine* 2019. doi:10.7326/M19-1326

26. Hooper L, et al. Reduction in saturated fat intake for cardiovascular disease. *Cochrane Database of Systematic Reviews* 2020. doi:10.1002/14651858.CD011737.pub3

27. Satija A, et al. Healthful and Unhealthful Plant-Based Diets and the Risk of Coronary Heart Disease in U.S. Adults. *J Am Coll Cardiol* 2017. doi:10.1016/j.jacc.2017.05.047

28. Dinu M, Abbate R, Gensini GF, Casini A, Sofi F. Vegetarian, vegan diets and multiple health outcomes: A systematic review with meta-analysis of observational studies. *Crit Rev Food Sci Nutr* 2017. doi:10.1080/10408398.2016.1138447

29. Nutrition, S. A. C. on. Saturated fats and health. (2019).

30. Health Canada. *Canada's Dietary Guidelines.* (2019).

31. Haider LM, Schwingshackl L, Hoffmann G, Ekmekcioglu C. The effect of vegetarian diets on iron status in adults: A systematic review and meta-analysis. *Crit Rev Food Sci Nutr* 2018. doi:10.1080/10408398.2016.1259210

32. Tong TYN, et al. Hematological parameters and prevalence of anemia in white and british indian vegetarians and nonvegetarians in the UK Biobank. *Am J Clin Nutr* 2019. doi:10.1093/ajcn/nqz072

33. Pawlak R, Berger J, Hines I. Iron Status of Vegetarian Adults: A Review of Literature. *Am J Lifestyle Med* 2018. doi:10.1177/1559827616682933

34. Fang X, et al. Dietary intake of heme iron and risk of cardiovascular disease: Adose-response meta-analysis of prospective cohort studies. *Nutr Metab Cardiovasc Dis* 2015. doi:10.1016/j.numecd.2014.09.002

35. Fonseca-Nunes A, Jakszyn P, Agudo, A. Iron and cancer risk-a systematic review and meta-analysis of the epidemiological evidence. *Cancer*

Epidemiology Biomarkers and Prevention 2014.
doi:10.1158/1055-9965.EPI-13-0733

36. Bao W, Rong Y, Rong S, Liu L. Dietary iron intake, body iron stores, and the risk of type 2 diabetes: A systematic review and meta-analysis. *BMC Med* 2012. doi:10.1186/1741-7015-10-119

37. Hurrell R, Egli I. Iron bioavailability and dietary reference values. *Am J Clin Nutr* 2010. doi:10.3945/ajcn.2010.28674F

38. Alves C, Saleh A, Alaofè H. Iron-containing cookware for the reduction of iron deficiency anemia among children and females of reproductive age in low- And middle-income countries: A systematic review. *PLoS One* 2019. doi:10.1371/journal.pone.0221094

39. Wagh K, et al. Lactase Persistence and Lipid Pathway Selection in the Maasai. *PLoS One* 2012. doi:10.1371/journal.pone.0044751

40. Mann GV, Shaffer RD, Anderson RS, Sandstead HH. Cardiovascular disease in the Maasai. *J Atheroscler Res* 1964. doi:10.1016/S0368-1319(64)80041-7

41. IARC. IARC Monographs evaluate consumption of red meat and processed meat. World Health Organization (2015). www.who.int/features/qa/cancer-red-meat/en/

42. WCRF. Diet, Nutrition, Physical Activity and Cancer: a Global Perspective. A summary of the Third Expert Report. (2018).

43. American College of Cardiology. Planting a Seed: Heart-Healthy Food Recommendations for Hospitals. American College of Cardiology. acc.org (2017).

44. Farvid MS, et al. Consumption of red and processed meat and breast cancer incidence: A systematic review and meta-analysis of prospective studies. *International J Cancer* 2018; 143: .

45. Li F, et al. Red and processed meat intake and risk of bladder cancer: A meta-analysis. *Int J Clin Exp Med* 2014; 7: .

46. Wolk A. Potential health hazards of eating red meat. *J Intern Med* 2017. doi:10.1111/joim.12543

47. Clinton SK, Giovannucci EL, Hursting SD. The World Cancer Research Fund/American Institute for Cancer Research Third Expert Report on Diet, Nutrition, Physical Activity, and Cancer: Impact and Future Directions. *J Nutrition* 2020; 150: .

48. GBD Diet Collaborators. Health effects of dietary risks in 195 countries, 1990–2017: a systematic analysis for the Global Burden of Disease Study 2017. *Lancet* 2019.

49. Gurjao C, et al. Discovery and features of an alkylating signature in colorectal cancer. *Cancer Discov* 2021. doi:10.1158/2159-8290.cd-20-1656

50. Bergeron N, Chiu S, Williams PT, King MS, Krauss RM. Effects of red meat, white meat, and nonmeat protein sources on atherogenic lipoprotein measures in the context of low compared with high saturated fat intake: a randomized controlled trial. *Am J Clin Nutr* 2019. doi:10.1093/ajcn/nqz035

51. Borgia L, et al. Long-termintake of animal flesh and risk of developing hypertension in three prospective cohort studies. *J Hypertens* 2015; 33: .

52. Song M, et al. Association of animal and plant protein intake with all-cause and cause-specific mortality. *JAMA Intern Med* 2016. doi:10.1001/jamainternmed.2016.4182

53. Sluijs I, et al. Dietary intake of total, animal, and vegetable protein and risk of type 2 diabetes in the European Prospective Investigation into Cancer and Nutrition (EPIC)-NL study. *Diabetes Care* 2010. doi:10.2337/dc09-1321

54. Rohrmann S, et al. Consumption of meat and dairy and lymphoma risk in the European Prospective Investigation into Cancer and Nutrition. *Int J Cancer* 2011. doi:10.1002/ijc.25387

55. Vergnaud AC, et al. Meat consumption and prospective weight change in participants of the EPIC-PANACEA study. *Am J Clin Nutr* 2010. doi:10.3945/ajcn.2009.28713

56. Carlsen MH, et al. The total antioxidant content of more than 3100 foods, beverages, spices, herbs and supplements used worldwide. *Nutr J* 2010. doi:10.1186/1475-2891-9-3

57. Miles FL, et al. Plasma, Urine, and Adipose Tissue Biomarkers of Dietary Intake Differ Between Vegetarian and Non-Vegetarian Diet Groups in the Adventist Health Study-2. *J Nutr* 2018. doi:10.1093/jn/nxy292

58. Zhang Q, Wang Y, Fu L. Dietary advanced glycation end-products: Perspectives linking food processing with health implications. *Compr Rev Food Sci Food Saf* 2020; 19: .

59. Uribarri J, et al. Dietary advanced glycation end products and their role in health and disease. *Advances in Nutrition* 2015; 6: .

60. Singh RK, et al. Influence of diet on the gut microbiome and implications for human health. *J Translational Med* 2017. doi:10.1186/s12967-017-1175-y

61. López-Moreno J, et al. Effect of Dietary Lipids on Endotoxemia Influences Postprandial Inflammatory Response. *J Agric Food Chem* 2017. doi:10.1021/acs.jafc.7b01909

62. Tang WHW, et al. Intestinal Microbial Metabolism of Phosphatidylcholine and Cardiovascular Risk. *N Engl J Med* 2013. doi:10.1056/NEJMoa1109400

63. Missailidis C, et al. Serum trimethylamine-N-Oxide is strongly related to renal function and predicts outcome in chronic kidney disease. *PLoS One* 2016. doi:10.1371/journal.pone.0141738

64. Heianza Y, et al. Long-Term Changes in Gut Microbial Metabolite Trimethylamine N-Oxide and Coronary Heart Disease Risk. *J Am Coll Cardiol* 2020. doi:10.1016/j.jacc.2019.11.060

65. Zhuang R, et al. Gut microbe–generated metabolite trimethylamine N-oxide and the risk of diabetes: A systematic review and dose-response meta-analysis. *Obesity Reviews* 2019. doi:10.1111/obr.12843

66. Jia J, et al. Assessment of causal direction between gut microbiota-

dependent metabolites and cardiometabolic health: A bidirectional mendelian randomization analysis. *Diabetes* 2019; 68: .

67. Mazidi M, Kengne A. Higher adherence to plant-based diets are associated with lower likelihood of fatty liver. *Clin Nutr* 2018.

68. Kahleova H, Levin S, Barnard N. Cardio-metabolic benefits of plant-based diets. *Nutrients* 2017. doi:10.3390/nu9080848

69. Levine ME, et al. Low protein intake is associated with a major reduction in IGF-1, cancer, and overall mortality in the 65 and younger but not older population. *Cell Metab* 2014. doi:10.1016/j.cmet.2014.02.006

70. Allen NE, et al. The associations of diet with serum insulin-like growth factor I and its main binding proteins in 292 women meat-eaters, vegetarians, and vegans. *Cancer Epidemiol Biomarkers Prev* 2002.

71. Barnard ND, Scialli AR, Hurlock D, Bertron P. Diet and sex-hormone binding globulin, dysmenorrhea, and premenstrual symptoms. *Obstet Gynecol* 2000. doi:10.1016/S0029-7844(99)00525-6

72. Ganmaa D, Cui X, Feskanich D, Hankinson SE, Willett WC. Milk, dairy intake and risk of endometrial cancer: A 26-year follow-up. *Int J Cancer* 2012. doi:10.1002/ijc.26265

73. Tabung FK, et al. Development and validation of an empirical dietary inflammatory index. *J Nutr* 2016. doi:10.3945/jn.115.228718

74. Messina M, Lynch H, Dickinson JM, Reed KE. No difference between the effects of supplementing with soy protein versus animal protein on gains in muscle mass and strength in response to resistance exercise. *Int J Sport Nutr Exerc Metab* 2018. doi:10.1123/ijsnem.2018-0071

75. Król W, et al. A vegan athlete's heart-is it different? Morphology and function in echocardiography. *Diagnostics* 2020. doi:10.3390/diagnostics10070477

76. Boutros GH, Landry-Duval MA, Garzon M, Karelis AD. Is a vegan diet detrimental to endurance and muscle strength? *Eur J Clin Nutr* 2020. doi:10.1038/s41430-020-0639-y

77. Hevia-Larraín V, et al. High-Protein Plant-Based Diet Versus a Protein-Matched Omnivorous Diet to Support Resistance Training Adaptations: A Comparison Between Habitual Vegans and Omnivores. *Sport Med* 2021; 2021.

78. Barnard ND, et al. Plant-based diets for cardiovascular safety and performance in endurance sports. *Nutrients* 2019. doi:10.3390/nu11010130

79. Kuchakulla M, Nackeeran S, Blachman-Braun R, Ramasamy R. The association between plant-based content in diet and testosterone levels in US adults. *World J Urol* 2020. doi:10.1007/s00345-020-03276-y

80. Allen NE, Appleby PN, Davey GK, Key TJ. Hormones and diet: low insulin-like growth factor-I but normal bioavailable androgens in vegan men. *Br J Cancer* 2002. doi:10.1054/bjoc.2000.1152

81. Kurniawan AL, Hsu CY, Rau HH, Lin LY, Chao JCJ. Dietary patterns in relation to testosterone levels and severity of impaired kidney function

among middle-aged and elderly men in Taiwan: A cross-sectional study. *Nutr J* 2019. doi:10.1186/s12937-019-0467-x

82. Maruyama K, Oshima T, Ohyama K. Exposure to exogenous estrogen through intake of commercial milk produced from pregnant cows. *Pediatr Int* 2010. doi:10.1111/j.1442-200X.2009.02890.x

83. Inman BA, et al. A population-based, longitudinal study of erectile dysfunction and future coronary artery disease. *Mayo Clin Proc* 2009. doi:10.4065/84.2.108

84. Ostfeld RJ, et al. Vasculogenic Erectile Dysfunction: The Impact of Diet and Lifestyle. *Am J Med* 2020. doi:10.1016/j.amjmed.2020.09.033

85. Aune D, et al. Dairy products, calcium, and prostate cancer risk: A systematic review and meta-analysis of cohort studies. *Am J Clin Nutr* 2015. doi:10.3945/ajcn.113.067157

86. Jacobsen BK, Knutsen SF, Fraser GE. Does high soy milk intake reduce prostate cancer incidence? The Adventist Health Study (United States). *Cancer Causes Control* 1998. doi:10.1023/A:1008819500080

87. Shin J, Millstine D, Ruddy B, Wallace M, Fields H. Effect of plant-and animal-based foods on prostate cancer risk. *J Am Osteopathic Assoc* 2019. doi:10.7556/jaoa.2019.123

88. ⬜rednicka-Tober, D. et al. Composition differences between organic and conventional meat: A systematic literature review and meta-analysis. *Br J Nutr* 2016. doi:10.1017/S0007114515005073

89. Vigar V, et al. A systematic review of organic versus conventional food consumption: Is there a measurable benefit on human health? *Nutrients* 2020; 12: .

90. Cohen Stuart J, et al. Comparison of ESBL contamination in organic and conventional retail chicken meat. *Int J Food Microbiol* 2012. doi:10.1016/j.ijfoodmicro.2011.12.034

91. Smith-Spangler C, et al. Are organic foods safer or healthier than conventional alternatives?: A systematic review. *Ann Intern Med* 2012. doi:10.7326/0003-4819-157-5-201209040-00007

92. Kesse-Guyot E, et al. Profiles of Organic Food Consumers in a Large Sample of French Adults: Results from the Nutrinet-Santé Cohort Study. *PLoS One* 2013. doi:10.1371/journal.pone.0076998

93. Lu C, et al. Organic diets significantly lower children's dietary exposure to organophosphorus pesticides. *Environ Health Perspect* 2006. doi:10.1289/ehp.8418

94. Baudry J, et al. Association of Frequency of Organic Food Consumption with Cancer Risk: Findings from the NutriNet-Santé Prospective Cohort Study. *JAMA Intern Med* 2018. doi:10.1001/jamainternmed.2018.4357

95. Bradbury KE, et al. Organic food consumption and the incidence of cancer in a large prospective study of women in the United Kingdom. *Br J Cancer* 2014. doi:10.1038/bjc.2014.148

96. Hall RH. A New Threat to Public Health: Organochlorines and Food. *Nutr Health* 1992. doi:10.1177/026010609200800103

References

97. Wu H, et al. Persistent organic pollutants and type 2 diabetes: A prospective analysis in the nurses' health study and meta-analysis. *Environmental Health Perspectives* 2013. doi:10.1289/ehp.1205248

98. Lim J, Park SH, Jee SH, Park H. Body concentrations of persistent organic pollutants and prostate cancer: a meta-analysis. *Environ Sci Pollut Res* 2015. doi:10.1007/s11356-015-4315-z

99. Park SH, Lim J, Park H, Jee SH. Body burden of persistent organic pollutants on hypertension: a meta-analysis. *Environ Sci Pollut Res* 2016: . doi:10.1007/s11356-016-6568-6

100. Hernández ÁR, et al. Consumption of organic meat does not diminish the carcinogenic potential associated with the intake of persistent organic pollutants (POPs). *Environ Sci Pollut Res* 2017. doi:10.1007/s11356-015-4477-8

101. Dervilly-Pinel G, et al. Micropollutants and chemical residues in organic and conventional meat. *Food Chem* 2017. doi:10.1016/j.foodchem.2017.04.013

102. Fraser AJ, Webster TF, McClean MD. Diet contributes significantly to the body burden of PBDEs in the general U.S. population. *Environ Health Perspect* 2009. doi:10.1289/ehp.0900817

103. Papadopoulou E, et al. Maternal diet, prenatal exposure to dioxins and other persistent organic pollutants and anogenital distance in children. *Sci Total Environ* 2013; 461–462: .

104. Bramwell L, et al. Predictors of human PBDE body burdens for a UK cohort. *Chemosphere* 2017; 189: .

105. Santo RE, et al. Considering Plant-Based Meat Substitutes and Cell-Based Meats: A Public Health and Food Systems Perspective. *Frontiers in Sustainable Food Systems* 2020; 4: .

106. Satija A, et al. Plant-Based Dietary Patterns and Incidence of Type 2 Diabetes in US Men and Women: Results from Three Prospective Cohort Studies. *PLoS Med.* (2016). doi:10.1371/journal.pmed.1002039

107. Hu FB, Otis BO, McCarthy G. Can Plant-Based Meat Alternatives Be Part of a Healthy and Sustainable Diet? *JAMA* 2019. doi:10.1001/jama.2019.13187

108. Crimarco A, et al. A randomized crossover trial on the effect of plant-based compared with animal-based meat on trimethylamine-N-oxide and cardiovascular disease risk factors in generally healthy adults: Study With Appetizing Plantfood—Meat Eating Alternative Trial (SWAP-ME. *Am J Clin Nutr* 2020. doi:10.1093/ajcn/nqaa203

109. Derbyshire E, Ayoob KT. Mycoprotein: Nutritional and Health Properties. *Nutr Today* 2019; 54: .

Chapter 3: Eating dairy

1. Michaëlsson K, et al. Milk intake and risk of mortality and fractures in women and men: Cohort studies. *Br Med J* 2014. doi:10.1136/bmj.g6015
2. Brondani JE, Comim FV, Flores LM, Martini LA, Premaor MO. Fruit and vegetable intake and bones: A systematic review and meta-analysis. *PLoS One* 2019. doi:10.1371/journal.pone.0217223
3. Willett WC, Ludwig DS. Milk and health. *New Eng J Med* 2020. doi:10.1056/NEJMra1903547
4. Storhaug CL, Fosse SK, Fadnes LT. Country, regional, and global estimates for lactose malabsorption in adults: a systematic review and meta-analysis. *Lancet Gastroenterol Hepatol* 2017. doi:10.1016/S2468-1253(17)30154-1
5. Price CT, Langford JR, Liporace FA. Essential Nutrients for Bone Health and a Review of their Availability in the Average North American Diet. *Open Orthop J* 2012; 6: .
6. Iguacel I, Miguel-Berges ML, Gómez-Bruton A, Moreno LA, Julián C. Veganism, vegetarianism, bone mineral density, and fracture risk: A systematic review and meta-analysis. *Nutr Rev* 2019. doi:10.1093/nutrit/nuy045
7. Tong TYN, et al. Vegetarian and vegan diets and risks of total and site-specific fractures: results from the prospective EPIC-Oxford study. *BMC Med* 2020. doi:10.1186/s12916-020-01815-3
8. Appleby P, Roddam A, Allen N, Key T. Comparative fracture risk in vegetarians and nonvegetarians in EPIC-Oxford. *Eur J Clin Nutr* 2007. doi:10.1038/sj.ejcn.1602659
9. Johansson H, et al. A meta-analysis of the association of fracture risk and body mass index in women. *J Bone Miner Res* 2014; 29: .
10. Davey GK, et al. EPIC–Oxford:lifestyle characteristics and nutrient intakes in a cohort of 33 883 meat-eaters and 31 546 non meat-eaters in the UK. *Public Health Nutr* 2003. doi:10.1079/phn2002430
11. Thorpe DL, Beeson WL, Knutsen R, Fraser GE, Knutsen SF. Dietary patterns and hip fracture in the Adventist Health Study 2: combined vitamin D and calcium supplementation mitigate increased hip fracture risk among vegans. *Am J Clin Nutr* 2021. doi:10.1093/ajcn/nqab095
12. Orlich MJ, et al. Vegetarian Epidemiology: Review and Discussion of Findings from Geographically Diverse Cohorts. *Adv Nutr* 2019. doi:10.1093/advances/nmy109
13. Health Canada. Canada's Dietary Guidelines. (2019).
14. Biban BG, Lichiardopol C. Iodine Deficiency, Still a Global Problem? *Curr Heal Sci J* 2017. doi:10.12865/CHSJ.43.02.01
15. Hetzel BS. The development of a global program for the elimination of brain damage due to iodine deficiency. *Asia Pacific J Clin Nutr* 2012; 21: .
16. van der Reijden OL, Zimmermann MB, Galetti V. Iodine in dairy milk:

References

Sources, concentrations and importance to human health. *Best Practice and Research: Clinical Endocrinology and Metabolism* 2017; 31: .

17. Levine ME, et al. Low protein intake is associated with a major reduction in IGF-1, cancer, and overall mortality in the 65 and younger but not older population. *Cell Metab* 2014. doi:10.1016/j.cmet.2014.02.006

18. Ji J, Sundquist J, Sundquist K. Lactose intolerance and risk of lung, breast and ovarian cancers: Aetiological clues from a population-based study in Sweden. *Br J Cancer* 2015. doi:10.1038/bjc.2014.544

19. Ganmaa D, Cui X, Feskanich D, Hankinson SE, Willett WC. Milk, dairy intake and risk of endometrial cancer: A 26-year follow-up. *Int J Cancer* 2012. doi:10.1002/ijc.26265

20. Youngman LD, Campbell TC. High protein intake promotes the growth of hepatic preneoplastic foci in Fischer #344 rats: Evidence that early remodeled foci retain the potential for future growth. *J Nutr* 1991. doi:10.1093/jn/121.9.1454

21. Khatami A, et al. Bovine Leukemia virus (BLV) and risk of breast cancer: A systematic review and meta-analysis of case-control studies. *Infectious Agents and Cancer* 2020; 15: .

22. Gao A, Kouznetsova VL, Tsigelny IF. Bovine leukemia virus relation to human breast cancer: Meta-analysis. *Microb Pathog* 2020; 149: .

23. Aune D, et al. Dairy products and colorectal cancer risk: A systematic review and meta-analysis of cohort studies. *Ann Oncology* 2012. doi:10.1093/annonc/mdr269

24. Aune D, et al. Dietary fibre, whole grains, and risk of colorectal cancer: Systematic review and dose-response meta-analysis of prospective studies. *BMJ Online* 2011. doi:10.1136/bmj.d6617

25. Aune D, et al. Dairy products, calcium, and prostate cancer risk: A systematic review and meta-analysis of cohort studies. *Am J Clin Nutr* 2015. doi:10.3945/ajcn.113.067157

26. Giovannucci E, Liu Y, Stampfer MJ, Willett WC. A prospective study of calcium intake and incident and fatal prostate cancer. *Cancer Epidemiol Biomarkers Prev* 2006; 15: .

27. Roddam AW, et al. Insulin-like growth factors, their binding proteins, and prostate cancer risk: Analysis of individual patient data from 12 prospective studies. *Ann Intern Med* 2008. doi:10.7326/0003-4819-149-7-200810070-00006

28. Allen NE, et al. The associations of diet with serum insulin-like growth factor I and its main binding proteins in 292 women meat-eaters, vegetarians, and vegans. *Cancer Epidemiol Biomarkers Prev* 2002.

29. Frattaroli J, et al. Clinical Events in Prostate Cancer Lifestyle Trial: Results From Two Years of Follow-Up. *Urology* 2008. doi:10.1016/j.urology.2008.04.050

30. Ornish D, et al. Effect of comprehensive lifestyle changes on telomerase activity and telomere length in men with biopsy-proven low-risk prostate cancer: 5-year follow-up of a descriptive pilot study. *Lancet Oncol* 2013; 14: .

31. Ornish D, et al. Changes in prostate gene expression in men undergoing an intensive nutrition and lifestyle intervention. *Proc Natl Acad Sci* 2008. doi:10.1073/pnas.0803080105

32. Mouzannar A, et al. Impact of Plant-Based Diet on PSA Level: Data From the National Health and Nutrition Examination Survey. *Urology* 2021. doi:10.1016/j.urology.2021.05.086

33. Wei Y, et al. Soy intake and breast cancer risk: a prospective study of 300,000 Chinese women and a dose–response meta-analysis. *Eur J Epidemiol* 2019. doi:10.1007/s10654-019-00585-4

34. Wang Q, Liu X, Ren S. Tofu intake is inversely associated with risk of breast cancer: A meta-analysis of observational studies. *PLoS One* 2020. doi:10.1371/journal.pone.0226745

35. Fraser GE, et al. Dairy, soy, and risk of breast cancer: those confounded milks. *Int J Epidemiol* 2020. doi:10.1093/ije/dyaa007

36. Korde LA, et al. Childhood soy intake and breast cancer risk in Asian American women. *Cancer Epidemiol Biomarkers Prev* 2009. doi:10.1158/1055-9965.EPI-08-0405

37. Applegate CC, Rowles JL, Ranard KM, Jeon S, Erdman JW. Soy consumption and the risk of prostate cancer: An updated systematic review and meta-analysis. *Nutrients* 2018. doi:10.3390/nu10010040

38. Juhl CR, et al. Dairy intake and acne vulgaris: A systematic review and meta-analysis of 78,529 children, adolescents, and young adults. *Nutrients* 2018. doi:10.3390/nu10081049

39. Murray MG, Kanuga J, Yee E, Bahna SL. Milk-induced wheezing in children with asthma. *Allergol Immunopathol (Madr)* 2013. doi:10.1016/j.aller.2012.07.002

40. Oranje AP, Wolkerstorfer A, De Waard-van der Spek FB. Natural course of cow's milk allergy in childhood atopic eczema/dermatitis syndrome. *Ann Allergy, Asthma and Immunol* 2002. doi:10.1016/S1081-1206(10)62123-0

41. Baseggio CA, Ierodiakonou D, Gowland MH, Boyle RJ, Turner PJ. Food anaphylaxis in the United Kingdom: Analysis of national data, 1998-2018. *Br Med J* 2021; 372: .

42. Morency ME, et al. Association between noncow milk beverage consumption and childhood height. *Am J Clin Nutr* 2017. doi:10.3945/ajcn.117.156877

43. Green J, et al. Height and cancer incidence in the Million Women Study: prospective cohort, and meta-analysis of prospective studies of height and total cancer risk. *Lancet Oncol* 2011. doi:10.1016/S1470-2045(11)70154-1

44. Ziegler EE. Consumption of cow's milk as a cause of iron deficiency in infants and toddlers. *Nutr Rev* 2011. doi:10.1111/j.1753-4887.2011.00431.x

45. Chia JSJ, et al. A1 beta-casein milk protein and other environmental pre-disposing factors for type 1 diabetes. *Nutr Diabetes* 2017. doi:10.1038/nutd.2017.16

46. Ludvigsson J. The jury is still out on possible links between cows' milk and type 1 diabetes. *Acta Paediatrica, International J Paediatrics* 2020. doi:10.1111/apa.14756

47. Vandenplas Y, et al. Safety of soya-based infant formulas in children. *Br J Nutrition* 2014. doi:10.1017/S0007114513003942

48. Rolim FRL, Freitas Neto OC, Oliveira MEG, Oliveira CJB, Queiroga RCRE. Cheeses as food matrixes for probiotics: In vitro and in vivo tests. *Trends in Food Science and Technology* 2020; 100: .

49. Valdes AM, Walter J, Segal E, Spector TD. Role of the gut microbiota in nutrition and health. *Br Med J* 2018. doi:10.1136/bmj.k2179

50. Tomova A, et al. The Effects of Vegetarian and Vegan Diets on Gut Microbiota. *Frontiers in Nutrition* 2019; 6: .

51. McDonald D, et al. American Gut: an Open Platform for Citizen Science Microbiome Research. *mSystems* 2018. doi:10.1128/msystems.00031-18

52. Septembre-Malaterre A, Remize F, Poucheret P. Fruits and vegetables, as a source of nutritional compounds and phytochemicals: changes in bioactive compounds during lactic fermentation. *Food Res Int* 2018; 104: .

53. James A, Wang Y. Characterization, health benefits and applications of fruits and vegetable probiotics. *CYTA - Journal of Food* 2019; 17: .

Chapter 4: Eating eggs

1. de Carvalho KMB, Pizato N, Botelho PB, Dutra ES, Gonçalves VSS. Dietary protein and appetite sensations in individuals with overweight and obesity: a systematic review. *Eur J Nutr* 2020. doi:10.1007/s00394-020-02321-1

2. Brennan IM, et al. Effects of fat, protein, and carbohydrate and protein load on appetite, plasma cholecystokinin, peptide YY, and ghrelin, and energy intake in lean and obese men. *Am J Physiol - Gastrointest Liver Physiol* 2012. doi:10.1152/ajpgi.00478.2011

3. Bayham BE, Greenway FL, Johnson WD, Dhurandhar NV. A randomized trial to manipulate the quality instead of quantity of dietary proteins to influence the markers of satiety. *J Diabetes Complications* 2014. doi:10.1016/j.jdiacomp.2014.02.002

4. Keogh JB, Clifton PM. Energy Intake and Satiety Responses of Eggs for Breakfast in Overweight and Obese Adults — A Crossover Study. *Int J Env Res Public Heal* 2020; 15: 5583.

5. Vander Wal JS, et al. Short-Term Effect of Eggs on Satiety in Overweight and Obese Subjects. *J Am Coll Nutr* 2005. doi:10.1080/07315724.2005.10719497

6. Lang V, et al. Satiating effect of proteins in healthy subjects: A comparison of egg albumin, casein, gelatin, soy protein, pea protein, and wheat gluten. *Am J Clin Nutr* 1998. doi:10.1093/ajcn/67.6.1197

7. Williamson DA, et al. Effects of consuming mycoprotein, tofu or chicken upon subsequent eating behaviour, hunger and safety. *Appetite* 2006; 46: .

8. Zhong VW, et al. Protein foods from animal sources, incident cardiovascular disease and all-cause mortality: A substitution analysis. *Int J Epidemiol* 2021; 50: ,

9. Réhault-Godbert S, Guyot N, Nys Y. The golden egg: Nutritional value, bioactivities, and emerging benefits for human health. *Nutrients* 2019. doi:10.3390/nu11030684

10. Huang J, et al. Association between Plant and Animal Protein Intake and Overall and Cause-Specific Mortality. *JAMA Intern Med* 2020. doi:10.1001/jamainternmed.2020.2790

11. Tang WHW, et al. Intestinal Microbial Metabolism of Phosphatidylcholine and Cardiovascular Risk. *N Engl J Med* 2013. doi:10.1056/NEJMoa1109400

12. Missailidis C, et al. Serum trimethylamine-N-Oxide is strongly related to renal function and predicts outcome in chronic kidney disease. *PLoS One* 2016. doi:10.1371/journal.pone.0141738

13. Heianza Y, et al. Long-Term Changes in Gut Microbial Metabolite Trimethylamine N-Oxide and Coronary Heart Disease Risk. *J Am Coll Cardiol* 2020. doi:10.1016/j.jacc.2019.11.060

14. Korde LA, et al. Childhood soy intake and breast cancer risk in Asian American women. *Cancer Epidemiol Biomarkers Prev* 2009. doi:10.1158/1055-9965.EPI-08-0405

15. Yang JJ, et al. Associations of choline-related nutrients with cardiometabolic and all-cause mortality: Results from 3 prospective cohort studies of blacks, whites, and Chinese. *Am J Clin Nutr* 2020. doi:10.1093/ajcn/nqz318

16. Koeth RA, et al. Intestinal microbiota metabolism of l-carnitine, a nutrient in red meat, promotes atherosclerosis. *Nat Med* 2013. doi:10.1038/nm.3145

17. The European Union One Health 2018 Zoonoses Report. *EFSA J* 2019. doi:10.2903/j.efsa.2019.5926

18. Thomas MK, et al. Estimates of Foodborne Illness – Related Hospitalizations. *Foodborne Pathog Dis* 2015; 12: .

19. Carson JAS, et al. Dietary cholesterol and cardiovascular risk: A science advisory from the American heart association. *Circulation* 2020. doi:10.1161/CIR.0000000000000743

20. Hooper L, et al. Reduction in saturated fat intake for cardiovascular disease. *Cochrane Database of Systematic Reviews* 2020. doi:10.1002/14651858.CD011737.pub3

21. Sacks FM, et al. Dietary fats and cardiovascular disease: A presidential advisory from the American Heart Association. *Circulation* 2017. doi:10.1161/CIR.0000000000000510

22. Bradbury KE, et al. Serum concentrations of cholesterol, apolipoprotein A-I and apolipoprotein B in a total of 1694 meat-eaters, fish-eaters, vegetarians and vegans. *Eur J Clin Nutr* 2014. doi:10.1038/ejcn.2013.248

23. Jenkins DJA, et al. Direct comparison of a dietary portfolio of cholesterol-lowering foods with a statin in hypercholesterolemic participants. *Am J Clin Nutr* 2005. doi:10.1093/ajcn.81.2.380

24. Khalighi Sikaroudi M, et al. The responses of different dosages of egg consumption on blood lipid profile: An updated systematic review and meta-analysis of randomized clinical trials. *J Food Biochem* 2020. doi:10.1111/jfbc.13263

25. Zhong VW, et al. Associations of Dietary Cholesterol or Egg Consumption with Incident Cardiovascular Disease and Mortality. *JAMA* 2019; 321: .

26. Zhuang P, et al. Egg and cholesterol consumption and mortality from cardiovascular and different causes in the United States: A population-based cohort study. *PLoS Med* 2021; 18: .

27. Wallin A, Forouhi NG, Wolk A, Larsson SC. Egg consumption and risk of type 2 diabetes: a prospective study and dose–response meta-analysis. *Diabetologia* 2016; 59: .

28. Drouin-Chartier JP,et al. Egg consumption and risk of cardiovascular disease: Three large prospective US cohort studies, systematic review, and updated meta-analysis. *Br Med J* 2020. doi:10.1136/bmj.m513

29. Shin JY, Xun P, Nakamura Y, He K. Egg consumption in relation to risk of cardiovascular disease and diabetes: A systematic review and meta-analysis. *Am J Clin Nutr* 2013; 98: .

30. Barnard ND, Long MB, Ferguson JM, Flores R, Kahleova H. Industry Funding and Cholesterol Research: A Systematic Review. *Am J Lifestyle Med* 2019. doi:10.1177/1559827619892198

Chapter 5: Eating fish

1. Li N, et al. Fish consumption and multiple health outcomes: Umbrella review. *Trends in Food Science and Technology* 2020. doi:10.1016/j.tifs.2020.02.033

2. Zhang B, Xiong K, Cai J, Ma A. Fish consumption and coronary heart disease: A meta-analysis. *Nutrients* 2020. doi:10.3390/nu12082278

3. Chowdhury R, et al. Association between fish consumption, long chain omega 3 fatty acids, and risk of cerebrovascular disease: Systematic review and meta-analysis. *Br Med J* 2012. doi:10.1136/bmj.e6698

4. Song M, et al. Association of animal and plant protein intake with all-cause and cause-specific mortality. *JAMA Intern Med* 2016. doi:10.1001/jamainternmed.2016.4182

5. Jayedi A, Shab-Bidar S. Fish Consumption and the Risk of Chronic Disease: An Umbrella Review of Meta-Analyses of Prospective Cohort Studies. *Advances in Nutrition* 2020; 11: .

6. Burr ML. Secondary prevention of CHD in UK men: The diet and

reinfarction trial and its sequel. *Proceedings of the Nutrition Society* 2007; 66: .

7. Burr ML, et al. Lack of benefit of dietary advice to men with angina: Results of a controlled trial. *Eur J Clin Nutr* 2003; 57: .

8. Mohan D, et al. Associations of Fish Consumption with Risk of Cardiovascular Disease and Mortality among Individuals with or without Vascular Disease from 58 Countries. *JAMA Intern Med* 2021; 181: .

9. Giem P, Beeson WL, Fraser GE. The incidence of dementia and intake of animal products: Preliminary findings from the Adventist Health Study. *Neuroepidemiology* 1993. doi:10.1159/000110296

10. Medawar E, Huhn S, Villringer A, Witte VA. The effects of plant-based diets on the body and the brain: a systematic review. *Translational Psychiatry* 2019. doi:10.1038/s41398-019-0552-0

11. Changzheng Y, et al. Dietary carotenoids related to risk of incident Alzheimer dementia (AD) and brain AD neuropathology: a community-based cohort of older adults. *Am J Clin Nutr* 2020; 113(1): 200-208. doi:10.1093/ajcn/nqaa303

12. Shishtar E, Rogers GT, Blumberg JB, Au R, Jacques PF. Long-term dietary flavonoid intake and risk of Alzheimer disease and related dementias in the Framingham Offspring Cohort. *Am J Clin Nutr* 2020. doi:10.1093/ajcn/nqaa079

13. Ramey MM, Shields GS, Yonelinas AP. Markers of a plant-based diet relate to memory and executive function in older adults. *Nutr Neurosci* 2020. doi:10.1080/1028415X.2020.1751506

14. Sabia S, et al. Association of ideal cardiovascular health at age 50 with incidence of dementia: 25 Year follow-up of Whitehall II cohort study. *Br Med J* 2019; 366: .

15. Hu Y, Hu FB, Manson JAE. Marine Omega-3 Supplementation and Cardiovascular Disease: An Updated Meta-Analysis of 13 Randomized Controlled Trials Involving 127 477 Participants. *J Am Heart Assoc* 2019; 8.

16. Abdelhamid AS, et al. Omega-3 fatty acids for the primary and secondary prevention of cardiovascular disease. *Cochrane Database of Systematic Reviews* 2020. doi:10.1002/14651858.CD003177.pub5

17. Sydenham E, Dangour AD, Lim WS. Omega 3 fatty acid for the prevention of cognitive decline and dementia. *Sao Paulo Med J* 2012. doi:10.1002/14651858.CD005379.pub3

18. Burckhardt M, et al. Omega-3 fatty acids for the treatment of dementia. Cochrane Database of Systematic Reviews. *Cochrane Database Syst Rev* 2016; 1: .

19. Bhatt DL, et al. Cardiovascular Risk Reduction with Icosapent Ethyl for Hypertriglyceridemia. *N Engl J Med* 2019. doi:10.1056/nejmoa1812792

20. Nicholls SJ, et al. Effect of High-Dose Omega-3 Fatty Acids vs Corn Oil on Major Adverse Cardiovascular Events in Patients at High Cardiovascular Risk. *JAMA* 2020.

21. Manson JE, et al. Marine n−3 Fatty Acids and Prevention of Cardiovascular Disease and Cancer. *N Engl J Med* 2019.

References

doi:10.1056/nejmoa1811403

22. Khan SU, et al. Effect of omega-3 fatty acids on cardiovascular outcomes: A systematic review and meta-analysis. *EClinicalMedicine* 2021. doi:10.1016/j.eclinm.2021.100997

23. Trichopoulou A, Bamia C, Trichopoulos D. Anatomy of health effects of Mediterranean diet: Greek EPIC prospective cohort study. *Br Med J* 2009. doi:10.1136/bmj.b2337

24. Wann LS, et al. Atherosclerosis in 16th-Century Greenlandic Inuit Mummies. *JAMA Netw Open* 2019. doi:10.1001/jamanetworkopen.2019.18270

25. Saini RK, Keum YS. Omega-3 and omega-6 polyunsaturated fatty acids: Dietary sources, metabolism, and significance — A review. *Life Sciences* 2018. doi:10.1016/j.lfs.2018.04.049

26. Burns-Whitmore B, Froyen E, Heskey C, Parker T, Pablo GS. Alpha-linolenic and linoleic fatty acids in the vegan diet: Do they require dietary reference intake/adequate intake special consideration? *Nutrients* 2019; 11: .

27. Simopoulos AP. The importance of the ratio of omega-6/omega-3 essential fatty acids. *Biomed Pharmacother* 2002; 56: .

28. Welch AA, Shakya-Shrestha S, Lentjes MAH, Wareham NJ, Khaw KT. Dietary intake and status of n-3 polyunsaturated fatty acids in a population of fish-eating and non-fish-eating meat-eaters, vegetarians, and vegans and the precursor-product ratio of α-linolenic acid to long-chain n-3 polyunsaturated fatty acids: Results. *Am J Clin Nutr* 2010. doi:10.3945/ajcn.2010.29457

29. Harris WS, et al. Blood n-3 fatty acid levels and total and cause-specific mortality from 17 prospective studies. *Nat Commun* 2021; 12: .

30. Craddock JC, Neale EP, Probst YC, Peoples GE. Algal supplementation of vegetarian eating patterns improves plasma and serum docosahexaenoic acid concentrations and omega-3 indices: a systematic literature review. *J Hum Nutr Diet* 2017; 30: .

31. Arterburn LM, et al. Algal-Oil Capsules and Cooked Salmon: Nutritionally Equivalent Sources of Docosahexaenoic Acid. *J Am Diet Assoc* 2008; 108: .

32. Statement on the benefits of fish/seafood consumption compared to the risks of methylmercury in fish/seafood. *EFSA J* 2015. doi:10.2903/j.efsa.2015.3982

33. Update of the monitoring of levels of dioxins and PCBs in food and feed. *EFSA J* 2012. doi:10.2903/j.efsa.2012.2832

34. Vendel AL, et al. Widespread microplastic ingestion by fish assemblages in tropical estuaries subjected to anthropogenic pressures. *Mar Pollut Bull* 2017. doi:10.1016/j.marpolbul.2017.01.081

35. Xue B, et al. Underestimated Microplastic Pollution Derived from Fishery Activities and 'Hidden' in Deep Sediment. *Environ Sci Technol* 2020. doi:10.1021/acs.est.9b04850

36. Ma Y, et al. The adverse health effects of bisphenol A and related toxicity

mechanisms. *Environl Res* 2019. doi:10.1016/j.envres.2019.108575

37. Donat-Vargas C, et al. Association between dietary intakes of PCBs and the risk of obesity: The SUN project. *J Epidemiol Community Health* 2014. doi:10.1136/jech-2013-203752

38. Silverstone AE, et al. Polychlorinated biphenyl (PCB) exposure and diabetes: Results from the Anniston community health survey. *Environ Health Perspect* 2012. doi:10.1289/ehp.1104247

39. Cohen L, Jefferies A. Environmental Exposures and Cancer: Using the Precautionary Principle. *Ecancermedicalscience* 2019. doi:10.3332/ecancer.2019.ed91

40. Starling P, Charlton K, McMahon AT, Lucas C. Fish intake during pregnancy and foetal neurodevelopment-A systematic review of the evidence. *Nutrients* 2015. doi:10.3390/nu7032001

41. Okocha RC, Olatoye IO, Adedeji OB. Food safety impacts of antimicrobial use and their residues in aquaculture. *Public Health Reviews* 2018. doi:10.1186/s40985-018-0099-2

42. Chen J, et al. Antibiotics and Food Safety in Aquaculture. *J Agric Food Chem* 2020; 68: 11908–11919.

43. Jacobs MN, Covaci A, Schepens P. Investigation of selected persistent organic pollutants in farmed Atlantic Salmon (Salmo salar), salmon aquaculture feed, and fish oil components of the feed. *Environ Sci Technol* 2002. doi:10.1021/es011287i

44. Lundebye AK, et al. Lower levels of Persistent Organic Pollutants, metals and the marine omega 3-fatty acid DHA in farmed compared to wild Atlantic salmon (Salmo salar). *Environ Res* 2017. doi:10.1016/j.envres.2017.01.026

Chapter 6: Eating fruit and vegetables

1. Jenkins DJA, et al. Effect of a very-high-fiber vegetable, fruit, and nut diet on serum lipids and colonic function. *Metabolism* 2001. doi:10.1053/meta.2001.21037

2. Aune D, et al. Fruit and vegetable intake and the risk of cardiovascular disease, total cancer and all-cause mortality—a systematic review and dose-response meta-analysis of prospective studies. *Int J Epidemiol* 2017; 46: 1029–1056.

3. Seidelmann SB, et al. Dietary carbohydrate intake and mortality: a prospective cohort study and meta-analysis. *Lancet Public Heal* 2018. doi:10.1016/S2468-2667(18)30135-X

4. Krssak M, et al. Intramyocellular lipid concentrations are correlated with insulin sensitivity in humans: A 1H NMR spectroscopy study. *Diabetologia* 1999. doi:10.1007/s001250051123

5. Sucharita S, et al. Evidence of higher intramyocellular fat among

References

normal and overweight Indians with prediabetes. *Eur J Clin Nutr* 2019. doi:10.1038/s41430-019-0402-4

6. Kantartzis K, et al. The lean insulin resistant phenotype. *Diabetes Pro* 2011; 1510-P.

7. Kahleova H, Falk Petersen K, Shulman GI, Shulman GI. Effect of a Low-Fat Vegan Diet on Body Weight, Insulin Sensitivity, Postprandial Metabolism, and Intramyocellular and Hepatocellular Lipid Levels in Overweight Adults. *JAMA Netw Open* 2020; 3(11): e2025454. doi: 10.1001/jamanetworkopen.2020.25454

8. Barnard ND, Cohen J, Jenkins DJA, et al. A low-fat vegan diet and a conventional diabetes diet in the treatment of type 2 diabetes: A randomized, controlled, 74-wk clinical trial. *Am J Clin Nutr* 2009; 89(5): 1588S-1596S. doi:10.3945/ajcn.2009.26736H

9. Li M, Fan Y, Zhang X, Hou W, Tang Z. Fruit and vegetable intake and risk of type 2 diabetes mellitus: meta-analysis of prospective cohort studies. *BMJ Open* 2014; 4(11): e005497. doi:10.1136/bmjopen-2014-005497

10. Zheng JS, Sharp SJ, Imamura F, et al. Association of plasma biomarkers of fruit and vegetable intake with incident type 2 diabetes: EPIC-InterAct case-cohort study in eight European countries. *Br Med J* 2020; 370: m2194. doi:10.1136/bmj.m2194

11. Christensen AS, Viggers L, Hasselström K, Gregersen S. Effect of fruit restriction on glycemic control in patients with type 2 diabetes--a randomized trial. *Nutr J* 2013; 12: 29. doi:10.1186/1475-2891-12-29

12. Du H, Li L, Bennett D, et al. Fresh fruit consumption in relation to incident diabetes and diabetic vascular complications: A 7-y prospective study of 0.5 million Chinese adults. *PLoS Med* 2017; 14(4): e1002279. doi:10.1371/journal.pmed.1002279

13. Papier K, Appleby PN, Fensom G, Knuppel A, et al. Vegetarian diets and risk of hospitalisation or death with diabetes in British adults: results from the EPIC-Oxford study. *Nutr Diabetes* 2019; 9(1): 7 doi: 10.1038/s41387-019-0074-0.

14. Toumpanakis A, Turnbull T, Alba-Barba I. Effectiveness of plant-based diets in promoting well-being in the management of type 2 diabetes: A systematic review. *BMJ Open Diabetes Research and Care* 2018; 6: e000534. doi:10.1136/bmjdrc-2018-000534

15. Kelly J, Karlsen M, Steinke G. Type 2 Diabetes Remission and Lifestyle Medicine: A Position Statement From the American College of Lifestyle Medicine. *Am J Lifestyle Med* 2020; 14(4): 406-419. doi: 10.1177/1559827620930962.

16. Donga E, Dekkers OM, Corssmit EPM, Romijn JA. Insulin resistance in patients with type 1 diabetes assessed by glucose clamp studies: Systematic review and meta-analysis. *Eur J Endocrin* 2015; 173(1): 101-109. doi:10.1530/EJE-14-0911

17. Priya G, Kalra S. A Review of Insulin Resistance in Type 1 Diabetes: Is

There a Place for Adjunctive Metformin? *Diabetes Therapy* 2018; 9: 349-361. doi:10.1007/s13300-017-0333-9

18. Kahleova H, Carlsen B, Berrien Lopez R, Barnard ND. Plant-Based Diets for Type 1 Diabetes. *J Diabetes Metab* 2020; 11(7): 847.

19. Clase CM, Carrero J-J, Ellison DH, et al. Potassium homeostasis and management of dyskalemia in kidney diseases: conclusions from a Kidney Disease: Improving Global Outcomes (KDIGO) Controversies Conference. *Kidney International* 2020; 97(1): 42-61. doi:10.1016/j.kint.2019.09.018

20. Joshi S, Hashmi S, Shah S, Kalantar-Zadeh K. Plant-based diets for prevention and management of chronic kidney disease. *Current Opinion in Nephrology and Hypertension* 2020; 29(1): 16-21. doi:10.1097/MNH.0000000000000574

21. Goraya N, Munoz-Maldonado Y, Simoni J, Wesson DE. Treatment of Chronic Kidney Disease-Related Metabolic Acidosis With Fruits and Vegetables Compared to NaHCO3 Yields More and Better Overall Health Outcomes and at Comparable Five-Year Cost. *J Ren Nutr* 2020; 31(3): 239-247. doi:10.1053/j.jrn.2020.08.001

22. Brunori G, Viola BF, Parrinello G, et al. Efficacy and Safety of a Very-Low-Protein Diet When Postponing Dialysis in the Elderly: A Prospective Randomized Multicenter Controlled Study. *Am J Kidney Dis* 2007; 49(5): 569-580. doi:10.1053/j.ajkd.2007.02.278

23. Joshi S, McMacken M, Kalantar-Zadeh K. Plant-Based Diets for Kidney Disease: A Guide for Clinicians. *Am J Kidney Diseases* 2021; 77: .

24. Guyton KZ, Loomis D, Grosse Y, et al. Carcinogenicity of tetrachlorvinphos, parathion, malathion, diazinon, and glyphosate. *Lancet Oncol* 2015; 16(5): 490-491. doi:10.1016/S1470-2045(15)70134-8

25. Bradbury KE, Balkwill A, Spencer EA, et al. Organic food consumption and the incidence of cancer in a large prospective study of women in the United Kingdom. *Br J Cancer* 2014; 110(9): 2321-2326. doi:10.1038/bjc.2014.148

26. Baudry J, Assmann KE, Touvier M, et al. Association of Frequency of Organic Food Consumption with Cancer Risk: Findings from the NutriNet-Santé Prospective Cohort Study. *JAMA Intern Med* 2018; 178(12): 1597-1606. doi:10.1001/jamainternmed.2018.4357

27. 't Mannetje A, De Roos AJ, Boffetta P, et al. Occupation and risk of non-hodgkin lymphoma and its subtypes: A pooled analysis from the interlymph consortium. *Environmental Health Perspectives* 2016; 124(4): 396-405. doi:10.1289/ehp.1409294

28. Rock CL, Thomson C, Gansler T, et al. American Cancer Society guideline for diet and physical activity for cancer prevention. *CA Cancer J Clin* 2020; 70(4): 245-271. doi:10.3322/caac.21591

29. Environmental Working Group. EWG's 2021 Shopper's Guide to Pesticides in Produce. 2021. www.ewg.org/foodnews/clean-fifteen.php. (Accessed 24 October 2021)

References

30. Mennella JA, Reiter AR, Daniels LM. Vegetable and fruit acceptance during infancy: Impact of ontogeny, genetics, and earlyexperiences. *Adv Nutr* 2016; 7(1): 211S-219S. doi: 10.3945/an.115.008649

31. Segovia-Siapco G, Burkholder-Cooley N, Tabrizi, SH, Sabaté J. Beyond meat: A comparison of the dietary intakes of vegetarian and non-vegetarian adolescents. *Front Nutr* 13 June2019. doi:10.3389/fnut.2019.00086

32. Verhage CL, Gillebaart M, van der Veek SMC, Vereijken CMJL. The relation between family meals and health of infants and toddlers: A review. *Appetite* 2018; 127: 97-109. doi: 10.1016/j.appet.2018.04.010.

33. McDonald D, Hyde E, Debelius JW, et al. American Gut: an Open Platform for Citizen Science Microbiome Research. *mSystems* 2018; 3(3). doi:10.1128/msystems.00031-18

34. Carlsen MH, Halvorsen BL, Holte K, et al. The total antioxidant content of more than 3100 foods, beverages, spices, herbs and supplements used worldwide. *Nutr J* 2010; 9: 3. doi:10.1186/1475-2891-9-3

35. Huang H, Chen G, Liao D, Zhu Y, Xue X. Effects of Berries Consumption on Cardiovascular Risk Factors: A Meta-analysis with Trial Sequential Analysis of Randomized Controlled Trials. *Sci Rep* 2016; 6: 23625. doi:10.1038/srep23625

36. Luís Â, Domingues F, Pereira L. Association between berries intake and cardiovascular diseases risk factors: A systematic review with meta-analysis and trial sequential analysis of randomized controlled trials. *Food and Function* 2018; 2. doi:10.1039/c7fo01551h

37. Hein S, Whyte AR, Wood E, Rodriguez-Mateos A, Williams CM. Systematic Review of the Effects of Blueberry on Cognitive Performance as We Age. *J Gerontol A Biol Sci Med Sci* 2019; 74(7): 984-995. doi:10.1093/gerona/glz082

38. Shishtar E, Rogers GT, Blumberg JB, Au R, Jacques PF. Long-term dietary flavonoid intake and risk of Alzheimer disease and related dementias in the Framingham Offspring Cohort. *Am J Clin Nutr* 2020; 112(2): 343-353. doi:10.1093/ajcn/nqaa079

39. Calvano A, Izuora K, Oh EC, et al. Dietary berries, insulin resistance and type 2 diabetes: An overview of human feeding trials. *Food Funct* 2019; 10. doi:10.1039/c9fo01426h

40. Royston KJ, Tollefsbol TO. The Epigenetic Impact of Cruciferous Vegetables on Cancer Prevention. *Current Pharmacology Reports* 2015; 1(1): 46-51. doi:10.1007/s40495-014-0003-9

41. Montgomery M, Srinivasan A. Epigenetic Gene Regulation by Dietary Compounds in Cancer Prevention. *Advances in Nutrition* 2019; 10(6): 1012-1028. doi:10.1093/advances/nmz046

42. Blekkenhorst LC, Prince RL, Ward NC, et al. Development of a reference database for assessing dietary nitrate in vegetables. *Mol Nutr Food Res* 2017; 61(8). doi: 10.1002/mnfr.201600982.

43. Bryan NS. Functional Nitric Oxide Nutrition to Combat Cardiovascular

Disease. *Current Atherosclerosis Reports* 2018; 20(5): 21. doi:10.1007/s11883-018-0723-0

44. Kapil V, Khambata RS, Robertson A, Caulfield MJ, Ahluwalia A. Dietary nitrate provides sustained blood pressure lowering in hypertensive patients: A randomized, phase 2, double-blind, placebo-controlled study. *Hypertension* 2015; 65(2): 320-327. doi:10.1161/HYPERTENSIONAHA.114.04675

45. Esselstyn CB, Gendy G, Doyle J, Golubic M, Roizen M. F. A way to reverse CAD? *J Fam Pract* 2014; 63(7): 356-364b. doi:10.1109/APUSNCURSINRSM.2017.8072476

46. Sakakibara S, Murakami R, Takahashi M, et al. Vinegar intake enhances flow-mediated vasodilatation via upregulation of endothelial nitric oxide synthase activity. *Biosci Biotechnol Biochem* 2010; 74(5): 1055-1061. doi:10.1271/bbb.90953

47. Bogdan C. Nitric oxide synthase in innate and adaptive immunity: An update. *Trends Immunol* 2015; 36(3): 161-178. doi:10.1016/j.it.2015.01.003

48. Jayachandran M, Xiao J, Xu B. A critical review on health promoting benefits of edible mushrooms through gut microbiota. *Int J Mol Sci* 2017; 18(9): 1934. doi:10.3390/ijms18091934

49. Ma G, Yang W, Zhao L, et al. A critical review on the health promoting effects of mushrooms nutraceuticals. *Food Sci Hum Wellness* 2018; 7(2): 125-133. doi:10.1016/j.fshw.2018.05.002

50. Ba DM, Ssentongo P, Beelman RB, et al. Higher Mushroom Consumption Is Associated with Lower Risk of Cancer: A Systematic Review and Meta-Analysis of Observational Studies. *Adv Nutr* 2021; 12(5): 1691-1704. doi:10.1093/advances/nmab015

51. Ba DM, Gao X, Muscat J, et al. Association of mushroom consumption with all-cause and cause-specific mortality among American adults: prospective cohort study findings from NHANES III. *Nutr J* 2021; 20(1): 38. doi: 10.1186/s12937-021-00691-8.

52. Stier H, Ebbeskotte V, Gruenwald J. Immune-modulatory effects of dietary Yeast Beta-1,3/1,6-D-glucan. *Nutr J* 2014; 13: 38. doi:10.1186/1475-2891-13-38

53. Wan Q, Li N, Du L, et al. Allium vegetable consumption and health: An umbrella review of meta-analyses of multiple health outcomes. *Food Sci Nutr* 2019; 7(8): 2451-2470. doi:10.1002/fsn3.1117

54. Sutliffe J, Scheid J, Gorman M, et al. Worksite Nutrition: Is a Nutrient-Dense Diet the Answer for a Healthier Workforce? *Am J Lifestyle Med* 2018; 12(5): 419-424. doi:10.1177/1559827618766485

55. Gerson M. The cure of advanced cancer by diet therapy: a summary of 30 years of clinical experimentation. *Physiol Chem Phys* 1978; 10(5): 449-464.

56. Hildenbrand GL, Hildenbrand LC, Bradford K, Cavin SW. Five-year survival rates of melanoma patients treated by diet therapy after the manner of Gerson: a retrospective review. *Altern Ther Health Med* 1995; 1(4): 29-37.

References

57. Molassiotis A, Peat P. Surviving against all odds: Analysis of 6 case studies of patients with cancer who followed the Gerson therapy. *Integr Cancer Ther* 2007; 6(1): 80-88. doi:10.1177/1534735406298258

58. Wei M, Brandhorst S, Shelehchi M, et al. Fasting-mimicking diet and markers/risk factors for aging, diabetes, cancer, and cardiovascular disease. *Sci Transl Med* 2017; 9(377): eaai8700. doi:10.1126/scitranslmed.aai8700

59. Henning SM, Yang J, Shao P, et al. Health benefit of vegetable/fruit juice-based diet: Role of microbiome. *Sci Rep* 2017; 7: 2167. doi:10.1038/s41598-017-02200-6

60. Rangan P, Choi I, Wei M, et al. Fasting-Mimicking Diet Modulates Microbiota and Promotes Intestinal Regeneration to Reduce Inflammatory Bowel Disease Pathology. *Cell Rep* 2019; 26(10): 2704-2719. doi:10.1016/j.celrep.2019.02.019

61. de Groot S, Lugtenburg RT, Cohen D, et al. Fasting mimicking diet as an adjunct to neoadjuvant chemotherapy for breast cancer in the multicentre randomized phase 2 DIRECT trial. *Nat Commun* 2020; 11(1): 3083. doi:10.1038/s41467-020-16138-3

62. Kim SY, Yoon S, Kwon SM, Park KS, Lee-Kim YC. Kale Juice improves coronary artery disease risk factors in hypercholesterolemic men. *Biomed Environ Sci* 2008; 21(2): 91-97. doi:10.1016/S0895-3988(08)60012-4

63. Kapil V, Khambata RS, Robertson A, Caulfield MJ, Ahluwalia A. Dietary nitrate provides sustained blood pressure lowering in hypertensive patients: A randomized, phase 2, double-blind, placebo-controlled study. *Hypertension* 2015; 65(2): 320-327. doi:10.1161/HYPERTENSIONAHA.114.04675

64. Butalla AC, Crane TE, Patil B, et al. Effects of a carrot juice intervention on plasma carotenoids, oxidative stress, and inflammation in overweight breast cancer survivors. *Nutr Cancer* 2012; 64(2): 331-341. doi:10.1080/01635581.2012.650779

65. Chazelas E, Srour B, Desmetz E, et al. Sugary drink consumption and risk of cancer: Results from NutriNet-Santé prospective cohort. *Br Med J* 2019; 366: 12408. doi:10.1136/bmj.12408

66. Auerbach BJ, Dibey S, Vallila-Buchman P, Kratz M, Krieger J. Review of 100% fruit juice and chronic health conditions: Implications for sugar-sweetened beverage policy. *Adv Nutr* 2018; 9(2): 78-85. doi:10.1093/advances/nmx006

Chapter 7: Eating whole grains

1. Aune D, Chan DSM, Lau R, et al. Dietary fibre, whole grains, and risk of colorectal cancer: Systematic review and dose-response meta-analysis of prospective studies. *BMJ Online* 2011; 343: d6617. doi:10.1136/bmj.d6617

2. Hullings AG, Sinha R, Liao LM, et al. Whole grain and dietary fiber intake and risk of colorectal cancer in the NIH-AARP Diet and Health Study cohort. *Am J Clin Nutr* 2020; 112(3): 6030612. doi:10.1093/ajcn/nqaa161

3. Aune D, Norat T, Romundstad P, Vatten LJ. Whole grain and refined grain consumption and the risk of type 2 diabetes: A systematic review and dose-response meta-analysis of cohort studies. *Eur J Epidemiol* 2013; 28(11): 845-858. doi:10.1007/s10654-013-9852-5

4. Aune D, Keum N, Giovannucci E, et al. Whole grain consumption and risk of cardiovascular disease, cancer, and all cause and cause specific mortality: Systematic review and dose-response meta-analysis of prospective studies. *Br Med J* 2016; 353: i2716. doi:10.1136/bmj.i2716

5. Mellen PB, Walsh TF, Herrington DM. Whole grain intake and cardiovascular disease: A meta-analysis. *Nutr Metab Cardiovasc Dis* 2008; 18(4): 283-290. doi:10.1016/j.numecd.2006.12.008

6. Marshall S, Petocz P, Duve E, et al. The Effect of Replacing Refined Grains with Whole Grains on Cardiovascular Risk Factors: A Systematic Review and Meta-Analysis of Randomized Controlled Trials with GRADE Clinical Recommendation. *J Acad Nutr Diet* 2020; 120(11): 1859-1883. doi:10.1016/j.jand.2020.06.021

7. Pletsch EA, Hamaker BR. Brown rice compared to white rice slows gastric emptying in humans. *Eur J Clin Nutr* 2018; 72(3): 367-373. doi:10.1038/s41430-017-0003-z

8. Holt SHA, Miller JC, Petocz P. An insulinindexof foods: the insulindemandgeneratedby 1000-kJ portions of common foods. *Am J Clin Nutr* 1997; 66(5): 1264-1276. doi: 10.1093/ajcn/66.5.1264.

9. Augustin LSA, Kendall CWC, Jenkins DJA, et al. Glycemic index, glycemic load and glycemic response: An International Scientific Consensus Summit from the International Carbohydrate Quality Consortium (ICQC). *Nutr Metab Cardiovasc Dis* 2015; 25(9): 795-815. doi:10.1016/j.numecd.2015.05.005

10. Berry S, Valdes A, Davies R, et al. Predicting Personal Metabolic Responses to Food Using Multi-omics Machine Learning in over 1000 Twins and Singletons from the UK and US: The PREDICT I Study (OR31-01-19). *Curr Dev Nutr* 2019; 3(1S). doi:10.1093/cdn/nzz037.or31-01-19

11. Jenkins DJA, Dehgan M, Mente A, et al. Glycemic Index, Glycemic Load, and Cardiovascular Disease and Mortality. *N Engl J Med* 2021; 384(14): 1312-1322. doi:10.1056/NEJMoa2007123

12. Mendosa D. Revised International Table of Glycemic Index (GI) and Glycemic Load (GL) Values—2008. *Living With Diabetes* 2008.

13. Foster-Powell K, Holt SHA, Brand-Miller JC. International table of gylcemic index and glycemic load values: 2002. *Am J Clin Nut.* 2002. doi:10.1093/ajcn/76.1.5

14. Bhavadharini B, et al. White rice intake and incident diabetes: A study of 132,373 participants in 21 countries. *Diabetes Care* 2020.

References

doi:10.2337/dc19-2335

15. Niland B, Cash BD. Health benefits and adverse effects of a gluten-free diet in non-celiac disease patients. *Gastroenterol Hepatol* 2018.
16. Czaja-Bulsa G, Bulsa M. What do we know now about IgE-mediated wheat allergy in children? *Nutrients* 2017. doi:10.3390/nu9010035
17. Barbaro MR, Cremon C, Stanghellini V, Barbara G. Recent advances in understanding non-celiac gluten sensitivity. *F1000Research* 2018. doi:10.12688/f1000research.15849.1
18. Dionne J, et al. A Systematic Review and Meta-Analysis Evaluating the Efficacy of a Gluten-Free Diet and a Low FODMAPs Diet in Treating Symptoms of Irritable Bowel Syndrome. *Am J Gastroenterol* 2018. doi:10.1038/s41395-018-0195-4
19. Fedewa A, Rao SSC. Dietary fructose intolerance, fructan intolerance and FODMAPs. *Curr Gastroenterol Rep* 2014; 16.
20. Taetzsch A, et al. Are gluten-free diets more nutritious? An evaluation of self-selected and recommended gluten-free and gluten-containing dietary patterns. *Nutrients* 2018. doi:10.3390/nu10121881
21. Vici G, Belli L, Biondi M, Polzonetti V. Gluten free diet and nutrient deficiencies: A review. *Clinical Nutrition* 2016. doi:10.1016/j.clnu.2016.05.002
22. Missbach B, et al. Gluten-free food database: The nutritional quality and cost of packaged gluten-free foods. *PeerJ* 2015. doi:10.7717/peerj.1337
23. Wu JHY, et al. Are gluten-free foods healthier than non-gluten-free foods? An evaluation of supermarket products in Australia. *Br J Nutr* 2015. doi:10.1017/S0007114515002056
24. Hanci O, Jeanes YM. Are gluten-free food staples accessible to all patients with coeliac disease? *Frontline Gastroenterol* 2019. doi:10.1136/flgastro-2018-101088
25. Potter MDE, Brienesse SC, Walker MM, Boyle A, Talley NJ. Effect of the gluten-free diet on cardiovascular risk factors in patients with coeliac disease: A systematic review. *J Gastroenterol Hepatol* 2018; 33(4): 781-791. doi:10.1111/jgh.14039
26. Lebwohl B, Cao Y, Zong G, et al. Long term gluten consumption in adults without celiac disease and risk of coronary heart disease: prospective cohort study. *Br Med J* 2017. doi:10.1136/bmj.j1892
27. Valvano M, Longo S, Stefanelli G, et al. Celiac disease, gluten-free diet, and metabolic and liver disorders. *Nutrients* 2020; 12(4): 940. doi:10.3390/nu12040940
28. Caio G, Lungaro L, Segata N, et al. Effect of gluten-free diet on gut microbiota composition in patients with celiac disease and non-celiac gluten/wheat sensitivity. *Nutrients* 2020; 12(6). doi:10.3390/nu12061832
29. Wang Y, Lebwohl B, Mehta R, et al. Long-term Intake of Gluten and Cognitive Function among US Women. *JAMA Netw Open* 2021; 4(5): e2113020. doi: 10.1001/jamanetworkopen.2021.13020.
30. Smith AH, Marshall G, Roh T, et al. Lung, bladder, and kidney cancer

mortality 40 years after arsenic exposure reduction. *J Natl Cancer Inst* 2018; 110(3): 241-249. doi:10.1093/jnci/djx201

31. Xu L, Polya DA, Li Q, Mondal D. Association of low-level inorganic arsenic exposure from rice with age-standardized mortality risk of cardiovascular disease (CVD) in England and Wales. *Sci Total Environ* 2020; 1743: 140534. doi:10.1016/j.scitotenv.2020.140534

32. Mitra A, Chatterjee S, Moogouei R, Gupta DK. Arsenic accumulation in rice and probable mitigation approaches: A review. *Agronomy* 2017; 7(4): 67. doi:10.3390/agronomy7040067

33. Thakur AK, Uphoff NT. How the system of rice intensification can contribute to climate-smart agriculture. *Agronomy J* 2017; 109(4): 1163-1182. doi:10.2134/agronj2016.03.0162

34. Majumder S, Banik P. Geographical variation of arsenic distribution in paddy soil, rice and rice-based products: A meta-analytic approach and implications to human health. *J Environ Management* 2019; 233: 184-199. doi: 10.1016/j.jenvman.2018.12.034.

35. Davis B, Melina V. *Becoming Vegan: Comprehensive Edition: The Complete Reference on Plant-based Nutrition*. 2014; Book Publishing Company.

36. Willett W, Rockstrom J, Loken B, et al. Food in the Anthropocene: the EAT–Lancet Commission on healthy diets from sustainable food systems. *Lancet* 2019; 393(10170): 447-492. doi: 10.1016/S0140-6736(18)31788-4.

37. WWF. *Future 50 Foods*. 2019. www.wwf.org.uk/sites/default/files/2019-02/Knorr_Future_50_Report_FINAL_Online.pdf (accessed 25 October 2021)

38. Rauber F, Louzada ML daC, Steele EM, et al. Ultra-processed foods and excessive free sugar intake in the UK: A nationally representative cross-sectional study. *BMJ Open* 2019; 9(10): e027546. doi:10.1136/bmjopen-2018-027546

39. Nardocci M, Leclerc B-S, Louzada M-L, et al. Consumption of ultra-processed foods and obesity in Canada. *Can J Public Heal* 2019; 110(1): 4-14. doi:10.17269/s41997-018-0130-x

40. Mazidi M, Katsiki N, Mikhailidis DP, Sattar N, Banach M. Lower carbohydrate diets and all-cause and cause-specific mortality: A population-based cohort study and pooling of prospective studies. *Eur Heart J* 2019; 40(34): 2870-2879. doi:10.1093/eurheartj/ehz174

41. Rosenbaum, M. et al. Glucose and Lipid Homeostasis and Inflammation in Humans Following an Isocaloric Ketogenic Diet. *Obesity* 2019; 27(6): 971-981. doi:10.1002/oby.22468

42. Kirkpatrick CF, Bolick JP, Kris-Ehterton PM, et al. Review of current evidence and clinical recommendations on the effects of low-carbohydrate and very-low-carbohydrate (including ketogenic) diets for the management of body weight and other cardiometabolic risk factors: A scientific statement from the Nati. *J Clin Lipidol* 2019; 13(5): 689-711. doi:10.1016/j.jacl.2019.08.003

43. The Scientific Advisory Committee on Nutrition. SACN report: lower

carbohydrate diets for type 2 diabetes. May 2021. https://assets. publishing.service.gov.uk/government/uploads/system/uploads/ attachment_data/file/1014673/SACN_report_on_lower_carbohydrate_ diets_for_type_2_diabetes.pdf

44. Gao, J. W. et al. Low-Carbohydrate Diet Score and Coronary Artery Calcium Progression: Results from the CARDIA Study. Arterioscler. Thromb. Vasc. Biol. (2020). doi:10.1161/ATVBAHA.120.314838

45. Anderson JW, Ward K. High-carbohydrate, high-fiber diets for insulin-treated men with diabetes mellitus. *Am J Clin Nutr* 1979; 32(11): 2312-2321. doi:10.1093/ajcn/32.11.2312

46. Jenkins DJA, Wong JMW, Kendall CWC, et al. Effect of a 6-month vegan low-carbohydrate ('Eco-Atkins') diet on cardiovascular risk factors and body weight in hyperlipidaemic adults: A randomised controlled trial. *BMJ Open* 2014; 4(2): e003505. doi:10.1136/bmjopen-2013-003505

Chapter 8: Eating beans and legumes

1. Noah ND, Bender AE, Reaidi GB, Gilbert RJ. Food poisoning from raw red kidney beans. *Br Med J* 1980; 281(6234): 236-237.

2. Lannoo N, Van Damme EJM. Lectin domains at the frontiers of plant defense. *Frontiers in Plant Science* 2014; 5: 397. doi:10.3389/fpls.2014.00397

3. Luo YW, Xie WH. Effect of different processing methods on certain antinutritional factors and protein digestibility in green and white faba bean (Vicia faba L.). *CYTA - J Food* 2013; 11(1): 43-49. doi:10.1080/19476337.2012.681705

4. Buettner D, Skemp S. Blue Zones: Lessons From the World's Longest Lived. *Am J Lifestyle Med* 2016; 10(5): 318-321. doi:10.1177/1559827616637066

5. Mazalovska M, Kouokam JC. Plant-Derived Lectins as Potential Cancer Therapeutics and Diagnostic Tools. *Biomed Res Int* 2020; 2020: 1631394. doi:10.1155/2020/1631394

6. Tröger W, Galun D, Reif M, et al. Viscum album [L.] extract therapy in patients with locally advanced or metastatic pancreatic cancer: A randomised clinical trial on overall survival. *Eur J Cancer* 2013; 49(18): 3788-3797. doi:10.1016/j.ejca.2013.06.043

7. Polak R, Phillips EM, Campbell A. Legumes: Health benefits and culinary approaches to increase intake. *Clin Diabetes* 2015; 33(4). doi:10.2337/diaclin.33.4.198

8. Naghshi S, Sadeghi O, Willett WC, Esmaillzadeh A. Dietary intake of total, animal, and plant proteins and risk of all cause, cardiovascular, and cancer mortality: Systematic review and dose-response meta-analysis of prospective cohort studies. *Br Med J* 2020; 370: m2412. doi:10.1136/bmj.m2412

9. Huang J, Liao LM, Weinstein SJ, et al. Association between Plant and Animal Protein Intake and Overall and Cause-Specific Mortality. *JAMA Intern Med* 2020; 180(9): 1173-1184. doi:10.1001/jamainternmed.2020.2790

10. Satija A, Malik V, Rimm, et al. Changes in intake of plant-based diets and weight change: Results from 3 prospective cohort studies. *Am J Clin Nutr* 2019; 110(3): 574-582. doi:10.1093/ajcn/nqz049

11. Satija A, Bhupathiraju SN, Rimm EB, et al. Plant-Based Dietary Patterns and Incidence of Type 2 Diabetes in US Men and Women: Results from Three Prospective Cohort Studies. *PLoS Med* 2016; 13(6): e1002039. doi:10.1371/journal.pmed.1002039

12. Li J, Mao Q-Q. Legume intake and risk of prostate cancer: A meta-analysis of prospective cohort studies. *Oncotarget* 2017; 8: 44776-44784. doi:10.18632/oncotarget.16794

13. Zhu B, Sun Y, Qi L, Zhong R, Miao X. Dietary legume consumption reduces risk of colorectal cancer: Evidence from a meta-analysis of cohort studies. *Sci Rep* 2015; 5: 8797. doi:10.1038/srep08797

14. Jenkins DJA, Kendall CWC, Augustin LSA, et al. Effect of legumes as part of a low glycemic index diet on glycemic control and cardiovascular risk factors in type 2 diabetes mellitus: A randomized controlled trial. *Arch Intern Med* 2012; 172(21): 1653-1560. doi:10.1001/2013.jamainternmed.70

15. Drewnowski A. The cost of US foods as related to their nutritive value. *Am J Clin Nutr* 2010; 92(5): 1181-1188. doi:10.3945/ajcn.2010.29300

16. Young VR. Soy protein in relation to human protein and amino acid nutrition. *J Am Dietetic Assoc* 1991; 91(7): 828-835.

17. Li N, Wu X, Xia L, et al. Soy and Isoflavone Consumption and Multiple Health Outcomes: Umbrella Review of Systematic Reviews and Meta-Analyses of Observational Studies and Randomized Trials in Humans. *Molecular Nutr Food Res* 2020; 64(4): 1900751. doi:10.1002/mnfr.201900751

18. Messina M, Mejia SB, Cassidy A, et al. Neither soyfoods nor isoflavones warrant classification as endocrine disruptors: a technical review of the observational and clinical data. *Critical Rev Food Sci Nutr* 27 March2021. doi:10.1080/10408398.2021.1895054

19. Messina M, Venter C. Recent Surveys on Food Allergy Prevalence. *Nutr Today* 2020; 55(1): 22-29. doi: 10.1097/NT.0000000000000389

20. MooreheadRA. Rodent models assessing mammary tumor prevention by Soy or Soy isoflavones. *Genes* 2019; 10(8): 566. doi:10.3390/genes10080566

21. Oseni T, Patel R, Pyle J, Jordan VC. Selective estrogen receptor modulators and phytoestrogens. *Planta Medica* 2008; 74(13): 1656-1665. doi:10.1055/s-0028-1088304

22. Korde LA, Wu AH, Fears T, et al. Childhood soy intake and breast cancer risk in Asian American women. *Cancer Epidemiol Biomarkers Prev* 2009; 18(4): 10501059. doi:10.1158/1055-9965.EPI-08-0405

23. Wang Q, Liu X, Ren S. Tofu intake is inversely associated with risk of breast cancer: A meta-analysis of observational studies. *PLoS One* 2020; 15(1): e0226745. doi:10.1371/journal.pone.0226745

References

24. Fraser GE, Jaceldo-Siegl K, Orlic M, et al. Dairy, soy, and risk of breast cancer: those confounded milks. *Int J Epidemiol* 2020; 49(5): 1526-1537. doi:10.1093/ije/dyaa007

25. Shu XO, Zheng Y, Cai H, et al. Soy food intake and breast cancer survival. *JAMA* 2009; 302(22): 2437-2443. doi: 10.1001/jama.2009.1783.

26. Akhlaghi M, Nasab MG, Riasatian M, Sadeghi F. Soy isoflavones prevent bone resorption and loss, a systematic review and meta-analysis of randomized controlled trials. *Critical Reviews in Food Science and Nutrition* 2020; 60(14): 2327-2341. doi:10.1080/10408398.2019.1635078

27. Nagata C, Takatsuka N, Kawakami N, Shimizu H. Soy product intake and hot flashes in Japanese women: Results from a community-based prospective study. *Am J Epidemiol* 2001; 153(8): 790-793. doi:10.1093/aje/153.8.790

28. Martinez J, Lewi JE. An unusual case of gynecomastia associated with soy product consumption. *Endocr Pract* 2008; 14(4): 415-418. doi:10.4158/EP.14.4.415

29. Reed KE, Camargo J, Hamilton-Reeves J, Kurzer M, Messina M. Neither soy nor isoflavone intake affects male reproductive hormones: An expanded and updated meta-analysis of clinical studies. *Reproductive Toxicology* 2021; 100: 60-67. doi: 10.1016/j.reprotox.2020.12.019.

30. Maruyama K, Oshima T, Ohyama K. Exposure to exogenous estrogen through intake of commercial milk produced from pregnant cows. *Pediatr Int* 2010; 52(1): 33-38. doi:10.1111/j.1442-200X.2009.02890.x

31. Michels KB, Binder N, Courant F, Franke AA, Osterhues A. Urinary excretion of sex steroid hormone metabolites after consumption of cow milk: A randomized crossover intervention trial. *Am J Clin Nutr* 2019; 109(2): 402-410. doi:10.1093/ajcn/nqy279

32. Applegate CC, Rowles JL, Ranard KM, Jeon S, Erdman JW. Soy consumption and the risk of prostate cancer: An updated systematic review and meta-analysis. *Nutrients* 2018; 10(1): 40. doi:10.3390/nu10010040

33. Jacobsen BK, Knutsen SF, Fraser GE. Does high soy milk intake reduce prostate cancer incidence? The Adventist Health Study (United States). *Cancer Causes Control* 1998; 9(6): 553-557. doi:10.1023/A:1008819500080

34. Dalais FS, Meliala A, Wattanapenpaiboon N, et al. Effects of a diet rich in phytoestrogens on prostate-specific antigen and sex hormones in men diagnosed with prostate cancer. *Urology* 2004; 64(3): 510-515. doi:10.1016/j.urology.2004.04.009

35. Pendleton JM, Tan WW, Anai S, et al. Phase II trial of isoflavone in prostate-specific antigen recurrent prostate cancer after previous local therapy. *BMC Cancer* 2008; 8: 132. doi:10.1186/1471-2407-8-132

36. Rizzo G, Baroni L. Soy, soy foods and their role in vegetarian diets. *Nutrients* 2018; 10(1): 43. doi:10.3390/nu10010043

37. Otun J, Sahebkar A, Östlundh L, Atkin SL, Sathyapalan T. Systematic Review and Meta-analysis on the Effect of Soy on Thyroid Function. *Sci*

Rep 2019; 9: 3964. doi:10.1038/s41598-019-40647-x

38. Messina M, Redmond G. Effects of soy protein and soybean isoflavones on thyroid function in healthy adults and hypothyroid patients: A review of the relevant literature. *Thyroid* 2006; 16(3): 249-258. doi:10.1089/thy.2006.16.249

39. Biban BG, Lichiardopol C. Iodine Deficiency, Still a Global Problem? *Curr Heal Sci J* 2017; 43(2): 103-111. doi:10.12865/CHSJ.43.02.01

40. Ford AC, Sperber AD, Corsetti M, Camilleri M. Irritable bowel syndrome. *Lancet* 2020; 396(10263): 1675-1688. doi:10.1016/S0140-6736(20)31548-8

41. Halmos EP, Gibson PR. Controversies and reality of the FODMAP diet for patients with irritable bowel syndrome. *J Gastroenterol Hepatol* 2019; 34(7): 1134-1142. doi:10.1111/jgh.14650

42. Caio G, Lungaro L, Segata N, et al. Effect of gluten-free diet on gut microbiota composition in patients with celiac disease and non-celiac gluten/wheat sensitivity. *Nutrients* 2020; 12(6). doi:10.3390/nu12061832

43. Desrochers N, Brauer PM. Legume Promotion in Counselling: An E-mail Survey of Dietitians. *Can J Diet Pract Res* 2001; 62(4): 193-198.

44. Doma KM, Farrell EL, Leith-Bailey ER, Soucier VD, Duncan AM. Motivators, Barriers and Other Factors Related to Bean Consumption in Older Adults. *J Nutr Gerontol Geriatr* 2019; 38(4): 397-413. doi:10.1080/21551197.2019.1646690

45. Qoueiroz K da S, de Oliveira AC, Helbig E, Reis SMPM, Carraro F. Soaking the common bean in a domestic preparation reduced the contents of raffinose-type oligosaccharides but did not interfere with nutritive value. *J Nutr Sci Vitaminol* 2002; 48(4): 283-289. doi:10.3177/jnsv.48.283

46. Oboh HA, Muzquiz M, Burbano C, et al. Effect of soaking, cooking and germination on the oligosaccharide content of selected Nigerian legume seeds. *Plant Foods Hum Nutr* 2000; 55(2): 97-110. doi:10.1023/A:1008133531726

47. Nkhata SG, Ayua E, Kamau EH, Shingiro J-B. Fermentation and germination improve nutritional value of cereals and legumes through activation of endogenous enzymes. *Food Sci Nutr* 2018; 6(8): 2446-2458. doi:10.1002/fsn3.846

48. Larijani B, Esfahani MM, Moghimi M, et al. Prevention and treatment of flatulence from a traditional Persian medicine perspective. *Iranian Red Crescent Med J* 2016; 18(4): e23664. doi:10.5812/ircmj.23664

Chapter 9: Eating nuts and seeds

1. Fraser GE, Sabate J, Beeson WL, Strahan TM. A Possible Protective Effect of Nut Consumption on Risk of Coronary Heart Disease: The Adventist Health Study. *Arch Intern Med* 1992; 152(7): 1416-1424. doi:10.1001/archinte.1992.00400190054010

References

2. Sabaté J, Fraser GE, Burke K, et al. Effects of Walnuts on Serum Lipid Levels and Blood Pressure in Normal Men. *N Engl J Med* 1993; 328(9): 603-607. doi:10.1056/nejm199303043280902

3. Becerra-Tomás N, Paz-Graniel I, Kendall CWC, et al. Nut consumption and incidence of cardiovascular diseases and cardiovascular disease mortality: A meta-analysis of prospective cohort studies. *Nutr Rev* 2019; 77(10): 691-709. doi:10.1093/nutrit/nuz042

4. Aune D, Keum N, Giovannucci E, et al. Nut consumption and risk of cardiovascular disease, total cancer, all-cause and cause-specific mortality: A systematic review and dose-response meta-analysis of prospective studies. *BMC Med* 2016; 14(1): 207. doi:10.1186/s12916-016-0730-3

5. Afshin A, Micha R, Khatibzadeh S, Mozaffarian D. Consumption of nuts and legumes and risk of incident ischemic heart disease, stroke, and diabetes: A systematic review and meta-analysis. *Am J Clin Nutr* 2014; 100(1): 278-288. doi:10.3945/ajcn.113.076901

6. Luo C, Zhang Y, Ding Y, et al. Nut consumption and risk of type 2 diabetes, cardiovascular disease, and all-cause mortality: A systematic review and meta-analysis. *Am J Clin Nutr* 2014; 100(1): 256-269. doi:10.3945/ajcn.113.076109

7. Liu G, Guasch-Ferre, Hu Y, et al. Nut Consumption in Relation to Cardiovascular Disease Incidence and Mortality among Patients with Diabetes Mellitus. *Circ Res* 2019; 124(6): 920-929. doi:10.1161/CIRCRESAHA.118.314316

8. Salas-Huetos A, Muralidharan J, Galiè S, Salas-Salvadó J, Bulló M. Effect of nut consumption on erectile and sexual function in healthy males: A Secondary outcome analysis of the fertinuts randomized controlled trial. *Nutrients* 2019; 11(6): 1372. doi:10.3390/nu11061372

9. Del Gobbo LC, Falk MC, Feldman R, Lewis K, Mozaffarian D. Effects of tree nuts on blood lipids, apolipoproteins, and blood pressure: Systematic review, meta-analysis, and dose-response of 61 controlled intervention trials. *Am J Clin Nutr* 2015; 102(6): 1347-1356. doi:10.3945/ajcn.115.110965

10. Ras RT, Geleijnse JM, Trautwein EA. LDL-cholesterol-lowering effect of plant sterols and stanols across different dose ranges: A meta-analysis of randomised controlled studies. *Br J Nutr* 2014; 112(2): 214-219. doi:10.1017/S0007114514000750

11. Smeets ETHC, Mensink RP, Joris PJ. Effects of tree nut and groundnut consumption compared with those of L-arginine supplementation on fasting and postprandial flow-mediated vasodilation: Meta-analysis of human randomized controlled trials. *Clin Nutr* 2021; 40(4): 1699-1710. doi:10.1016/j.clnu.2020.09.015

12. Neale EP, Tapsell LC, Guan V, Batterham MJ. The effect of nut consumption on markers of inflammation and endothelial function: A systematic review and meta-analysis of randomised controlled trials. *BMJ Open* 2017; 7: e016863. doi:10.1136/bmjopen-2017-016863

13. Viguiliouk E, Kendall CWC, Mejia SB, et al. Effect of tree nuts on glycemic control in diabetes: A systematic review and meta-analysis of randomized controlled dietary trials. *PLoS One* 2014; 9(7): e103376. doi:10.1371/journal.pone.0103376

14. Tindall AM, Johnston EA, Kris-Etherton PM, Petersen KS. The effect of nuts on markers of glycemic control: A systematic review and meta-Analysis of randomized controlled trials. *Am J Clin Nutr* 2019; 109(2): 297-314. doi:10.1093/ajcn/nqy236

15. Bolling BW, McKay DL, Blumberg JB. The phytochemical composition and antioxidant actions of tree nuts. *Asia Pac J Clin Nutr* 2010; 19(1): 117-123. PMCID: PMC5012104

16. De Souza RGM, Schincaglia RM, Pimentel GD, Mota JF. Nuts and human health outcomes: A systematic review. *Nutrients* 2017; 9(12): 1311. doi:10.3390/nu9121311

17. Sacks FM, Lichtenstein AH, Wu JHY, et al. Dietary fats and cardiovascular disease: A presidential advisory from the American Heart Association. *Circulation* 2017; 136: e1-e23. doi:10.1161/CIR.0000000000000510

18. Tan SY, Dhillon J, Mattes RD. A review of the effects of nuts on appetite, food intake, metabolism, and body weight. *Am J Clin Nutr* 2014; 100(S1): 412S-1422S. doi:10.3945/ajcn.113.071456

19. Liu X, Li Y, Guasch-Ferre M, et al. Changes in nut consumption influence long-term weight change in US men and women. *BMJ Nutr Prev Heal* 2019; 0: 1-10. doi:10.1136/bmjnph-2019-000034

20. Jackson CL, Hu FB. Long-term associations of nut consumption with body weight and obesity. *Am J Clin Nutr* 2014; 100(S1): 408S-411S. doi:10.3945/ajcn.113.071332

21. Fitzgerald E, Lambert K, Stanford J, Neale EP. The effect of nut consumption (tree nuts and peanuts) on the gut microbiota of humans: A systematic review. *Br J Nutr* 2020; 125(5): 508-520. doi:10.1017/S0007114520002925

22. Guasch-Ferré M, Liu X, Malik VS, et al. Nut Consumption and Risk of Cardiovascular Disease. *J Am Coll Cardiol* 2017; 70(20): 2519-2532. doi:10.1016/j.jacc.2017.09.035

23. Chaddha A, Eagle KA. Omega-3 Fatty Acids and Heart Health. *Circulation* 2015; 132: e350-e352. doi:10.1161/CIRCULATIONAHA.114.015176

24. Pan A, Sun Q, Manson JAE, Willett WC, Hu FB. Walnut consumption is associated with lower risk of type 2 diabetes in women. *J Nutr* 2013; 143(4): 512-518. doi:10.3945/jn.112.172171

25. Cofán M, Rajaram S, Sala-Vila A, et al. Effects of 2-Year Walnut-Supplemented Diet on Inflammatory Biomarkers. *J Am Coll Cardiol* 2020; 76(19): 2282-2284. doi:10.1016/j.jacc.2020.07.071

26. Ros E, Rajaram S, Sala-Vila A, et al. Effect of a 1-year walnut supplementation on blood lipids among older individuals: Findings from the walnuts and healthy aging (WAHA) study. *FASEB Journal* 2016; 30(2).

References

www.cochranelibrary.com/central/doi/10.1002/central/CN-01266498/full

27. Katz DL, Davidhi A, Ma Y, et al. Effects of walnuts on endothelial function in overweight adults with visceral obesity: a randomized, controlled, crossover trial. *J Am Coll Nutr* 2012; 31(6): 415-423. doi:10.1080/07315724.2012.10720468

28. Burbank AJ, Duran CG, Pan Y, et al. Gamma tocopherol-enriched supplement reduces sputum eosinophilia and endotoxin-induced sputum neutrophilia in volunteers with asthma. *J Allergy Clin Immunol* 2018; 141(4): 1231-1238. doi:10.1016/j.jaci.2017.06.029

29. Chauhan A, Chauhan V. Beneficial effects of walnuts on cognition and brain health. *Nutrients* 2020; 12(2): 550. doi:10.3390/nu12020550

30. Sala-Vila A, Valls-Pedret C, Rajaram S, Coll-Padros N. Effect of a 2-year diet intervention with walnuts on cognitive decline. The Walnuts and Healthy Aging (WAHA) study: a randomized controlled trial. *Am J Clin Nutr* 2020; 111(S4): 1-11. doi:10.1093/ajcn/nqz328

31. Stiefel G, Anagnostou K, Boyle RJ, et al. BSACI guideline for the diagnosis and management of peanut and tree nut allergy. *Clin Exp Allergy* 2017; 47: 719-739. doi:10.1111/cea.12957

32. Du Toit G, Roberts G, Sayre PH, et al. Randomized Trial of Peanut Consumption in Infants at Risk for Peanut Allergy. *N Engl J Med* 2015; 372(9): 803-813. doi:10.1056/nejmoa1414850

33. Gupta RS, Bilaver LA, Johnson JL, et al. Assessment of Pediatrician Awareness and Implementation of the Addendum Guidelines for the Prevention of Peanut Allergy in the United States. *JAMA Netw Open* 2020; 3(7): e2010511. doi:10.1001/jamanetworkopen.2020.10511

34. Parikh M, Maddaford TG, Austria JA, et al. Dietary flaxseed as a strategy for improving human health. *Nutrients* 2019; 11(5): 1171. doi:10.3390/nu11051171

35. Rodriguez-Leyva D, Weighell W, Edel AL, et al. Potent antihypertensive action of dietary flaxseed in hypertensive patients. *Hypertension* 2013; 62(6): 1081-1089. doi:10.1161/HYPERTENSIONAHA.113.02094

36. Caligiuri SPB, Aukema HM, Ravandi A, et al. Flaxseed consumption reduces blood pressure in patients with hypertension by altering circulating oxylipins via an α-linolenic acid-induced inhibition of soluble epoxide hydrolase. *Hypertension* 2014; 64(1): 53-59. doi:10.1161/HYPERTENSIONAHA.114.03179

37. Soltanian N, Janghorbani M. A randomized trial of the effects of flaxseed to manage constipation, weight, glycemia, and lipids in constipated patients with type 2 diabetes. *Nutr Metab* 2018; 15: 36. doi:10.1186/s12986-018-0273-z

38. Flower G, Fritz H, Balneaves LG. Flax and breast cancer: A systematic review. *Integrative Cancer Therapies* 2014; 13(3): 181-192. doi:10.1177/1534735413502076

39. Demark-Wahnefried W, Polascik TJ, George SL, et al. Flaxseed

supplementation (not dietary fat restriction) reduces prostate cancer proliferation rates in men presurgery. *Cancer Epidemiol Biomarkers Prev* 2008; 17(12): 3577-3587. doi:10.1158/1055-9965.EPI-08-0008

40. Lesser LI, Ebbeling CB, Goozner M, Wypij D, Ludwig DS. Relationship between funding source and conclusion among nutrition-related scientific articles. *PLoS Med* 2007; 4(1): e5. doi:10.1371/journal.pmed.0040005

41. Li N, Jia X, Chen C-YO, et al. Almond consumption reduces oxidative DNA damage and lipid peroxidation in male smokers. *J Nutr* 2007; 137(12); 2717-2722. doi:10.1093/jn/137.12.2717

42. Nestle M. Food industry funding of nutrition research: The relevance of history for current debates. *JAMA Internal Medicine* 2016; 176(1): 13-14. doi:10.1001/jamainternmed.2016.5400

43. Nestle M. Corporate funding of food and nutrition research science or marketing? *JAMA Internal Medicine* 2016; 176(1): 13-14. doi:10.1001/jamainternmed.2015.6667

Chapter 10: Foods and nutrients of special interest

1. Freeman AM, Morris PB, Barnard N, et al. Trending Cardiovascular Nutrition Controversies. *J Am Coll Cardiol* 2017; 69(9): 1172-1187. doi:10.1016/j.jacc.2016.10.086

2. Nocella C, Cammisotto V, Fianchini L, et al. Extra Virgin Olive Oil and Cardiovascular Diseases: Benefits for Human Health. *Endocr Metab Immune Disord Drug Targets* 2017; 18(1): 4-13. doi:10.2174/1871530317666171114121533

3. Ghobadi S, Hassanzadeh-Rostami Z, Mohammadian F, et al. Comparison of blood lipid-lowering effects of olive oil and other plant oils: A systematic review and meta-analysis of 27 randomized placebo-controlled clinical trials. *Critical Rev Food Sci Nutr* 2019; 59(13). doi:10.1080/10408398.2018.1438349

4. Tsartsou E, Proutsos N, Castanas E, Kampa M. Network meta-analysis of metabolic effects of olive-oil in humans shows the importance of olive oil consumption with moderate polyphenol levels as part of the Mediterranean diet. *Front Nutr* 2019; 6: 6. doi:10.3389/fnut.2019.00006

5. European Food Safety Authority. Scientific Opinion on the substantiation of health claims related to olive oil and maintenance of normal blood LDL-cholesterol concentrations (ID 1316, 1332), maintenance of normal (fasting) blood concentrations of triglycerides (ID 1316, 1332), maintenan. *EFSA J* 2011; 9(4): 2044. doi:10.2903/j.efsa.2011.2044

6. EFSA Panel on Dietetic Products, Nutrition and Allergies. Scientific Opinion on the substantiation of a health claim related to polyphenols in olive and maintenance of normal blood HDL cholesterol concentrations

References

(ID 1639, further assessment) pursuant to Article 13(1) of Regulation (EC) No 1924/2006. *EFSA J* 2012; 10(8): 2848. doi:10.2903/j.efsa.2012.2848

7. Rueda-Clausen CF, Silva FA, Lindarte MA, et al. Olive, soybean and palm oils intake have a similar acute detrimental effect over the endothelial function in healthy young subjects. *Nutr Metab Cardiovasc Dis* 2007; 17(1): 50-57. doi:10.1016/j.numecd.2005.08.008

8. Schwingshackl L, Christoph M, Hoffmann G. Effects of olive oil on markers of inflammation and endothelial function—A systematic review and meta-analysis. *Nutrients* 2015; 7(9). doi:10.3390/nu7095356

9. Pérez-Jiménez J, Neveu V, Vos F, Scalbert A. Identification of the 100 richest dietary sources of polyphenols: An application of the Phenol-Explorer database. *Eur J Clin Nutr* 2010; 64: S112-S120. doi:10.1038/ejcn.2010.221

10. Kaplan H, Thompson RC, Trumble C, et al. Coronary atherosclerosis in indigenous South American Tsimane: a cross-sectional cohort study. *Lancet* 2017; 389(10080): 1730-1739. doi:10.1016/S0140-6736(17)30752-3

11. Willcox DC, Scapagnini G, Willcox BJ. Healthy aging diets other than the Mediterranean: A focus on the Okinawan diet. *Mech Ageing Dev* 2014; 136-137: 148-162. doi:10.1016/j.mad.2014.01.002

12. Amiri M, Raeisi-Dehkordi H, Sarrafzadegan N, Forbes SC, Salehi-Abargouei A. The effects of Canola oil on cardiovascular risk factors: A systematic review and meta-analysis with dose-response analysis of controlled clinical trials. *Nutr Metab Cardiovasc Dis* 2020; 30(12): 2133-2145. doi:10.1016/j.numecd.2020.06.007

13. Neelakantan N, Seah JYH, van Dam RM. The Effect of Coconut Oil Consumption on Cardiovascular Risk Factors: A Systematic Review and Meta-Analysis of Clinical Trials. *Circulation* 2020; 141(10): 803-814. doi:10.1161/CIRCULATIONAHA.119.043052

14. Landmesser U, Hazen S. HDL-cholesterol, genetics, and coronary artery disease: The myth of the 'good cholesterol'? *Eur Heart J* 2018; 39(23): 2179-2182. doi:10.1093/eurheartj/ehy299

15. EFSA. Scientific Opinion on the use of cobalt compounds as additives in animal nutrition. *EFSA J* 2009; 7(12): 1383. doi:10.2903/j.efsa.2009.1383

16. DSM Vitamin Supplementation Guidelines 2011 for domestic animals. 12th edition. www.dsm.com/content/dam/dsm/anh/en_US/documents/OVN_supplementation_guidelines.pdf (accessed 26 October 2021)

17. Stover PJ. Vitamin B12 and older adults. *Curr Opin Clin Nutr Metab Care* 2010; 13(1): 24-27. doi:10.1097/MCO.0b013e328333d157

18. NIH Office of Dietary Supplements. Vitamin B-12 Fact Sheet for Health Professionals. Advances in Nutrition (2018). https://ods.od.nih.gov/factsheets/VitaminB12-HealthProfessional/ (accessed 26 October 2021)

19. Tucker KL, Rich S, Rosenberg, et al. Plasma vitamin B-12 concentrations relate to intake source in the framingham offspring study. *Am J Clin Nutr* 2000; 71(2): 514-522. doi: 10.1093/ajcn/71.2.514.

20. Kaplan A, Zelicha H, Tsaban G, et al. Protein bioavailability of Wolffia

globosa duckweed, a novel aquatic plant – A randomized controlled trial. *Clin Nutr* 2019; 38(6): 2576-2582. doi:10.1016/j.clnu.2018.12.009

21. Tsaban G, Meir AY, Rinott E, et al. The effect of green Mediterranean diet on cardiometabolic risk; A randomised controlled trial. *Heart* 2020; 317802. doi:10.1136/heartjnl-2020-317802

22. Meir AY, Rinott E, Tsaban G, et al. Effect of green-Mediterranean diet on intrahepatic fat: the DIRECT PLUS randomised controlled trial. *Gut* 2021; 70(11): 2085-2095. doi:10.1136/gutjnl-2020-323106

23. Herrmann W, Obeid R, Schorr H, Geisel J. The Usefulness of Holotranscobalamin in Predicting Vitamin B12 Status in Different Clinical Settings. *Curr Drug Metab* 2005; 6(1): 47-53. doi: 10.2174/1389200052997384.

24. Zugravu C-A, Macri A, Belc N, Bohiltea R. Efficacy of supplementation with methylcobalamin and cyancobalamin in maintaining the level of serum holotranscobalamin in a group of plant-based diet (vegan) adults. *Exp Ther Med* 2021; 22(3): 993. doi:10.3892/etm.2021.10425

25. Del Bo C, Riso P, Gardana C, et al. Effect of two different sublingual dosages of vitamin B 12 on cobalamin nutritional status in vegans and vegetarians with a marginal deficiency: A randomized controlled trial. *Clin Nutr* 2019; 38(2): 575-583. doi: 10.1016/j.clnu.2018.02.008

26. Abdulwaliyu I, Arekemase SO, Adudu JA, et al. Investigation of the medicinal significance of phytic acid as an indispensable anti-nutrient in diseases. *Clin Nutr Experimental* 2019; 28: 42-61. doi:10.1016/j.yclnex.2019.10.002

27. Davey GK, Spencer EA, Appleby PN, Allen NE, Knox KH, Key TJ. EPIC–Oxford:lifestyle characteristics and nutrient intakes in a cohort of 33 883 meat-eaters and 31 546 non meat-eaters in the UK. *Public Health Nutr* 2003; 6(3): 259-269. doi:10.1079/phn2002430

28. Rizzo NS, Jaceldo-Siegl K, Sabate J, Fraser GE. Nutrient Profiles of Vegetarian and Nonvegetarian Dietary Patterns. *J Acad Nutr Diet* 2013; 113(12): 1610-1619. doi:10.1016/j.jand.2013.06.349

29. Foster M, Chu A, Petocz P, Samman S. Effect of vegetarian diets on zinc status: A systematic review and meta-analysis of studies in humans. *J Sci Food Agriculture* 2013; 93(10): 2362-2371. doi:10.1002/jsfa.6179

30. Foster M, Herulah UN, Prasad A, Petocz P, Samman S. Zinc status of vegetarians during pregnancy: A systematic review of observational studies and meta-analysis of zinc intake. *Nutrients* 2015. doi:10.3390/nu7064512

31. Dawson, M. The Importance of Vitamin A in Nutrition. *Curr Pharm Des* 2005. doi:10.2174/1381612003401190

32. Borel P, Desmarchelier C. Genetic variations associated with vitamin a status and vitamin A bioavailability. *Nutrients* 2017. doi:10.3390/nu9030246

33. Kopec RE, et al. Avocado consumption enhances human postprandial provitamin a absorption and conversion from a novel high-β-carotene

References

tomato sauce and from carrots. *J Nutr* 2014. doi:10.3945/jn.113.187674

34. Derbyshire E. Could we be overlooking a potential choline crisis in the United Kingdom? *BMJ Nutr Prev Heal* 2019; 0: 1-4. doi:10.1136/bmjnph-2019-000037

35. Giem P, Beeson WL, Fraser GE. The incidence of dementia and intake of animal products: Preliminary findings from the Adventist Health Study. *Neuroepidemiology* 1993; 12(1): 28-36. doi:10.1159/000110296

36. Health N. I. of Choline Fact Sheet for Health Professionals. *Office of Dietary Supplements* 2019.

37. EFSA Panel on Dietetic Products, Nutrition and Allergies (NDA). Dietary Reference Values for choline. *EFSA J* 2016; 14(8): 4484. doi:10.2903/j.efsa.2016.4484

38. Tang WHW, Wang Z, Levison BS, et al. Intestinal Microbial Metabolism of Phosphatidylcholine and Cardiovascular Risk. *N Engl J Med* 2013; 368: 1575-1584. doi:10.1056/NEJMoa1109400

39. Zhuang R, Ge X, Han L, et al. Gut microbe–generated metabolite trimethylamine N-oxide and the risk of diabetes: A systematic review and dose-response meta-analysis. *Obesity Reviews* 2019; 20(6): 883-894. doi:10.1111/obr.12843

40. Farhangi MA, Vajdi M, Asghari-Jafarabadi M. Gut microbiota-Associated metabolite trimethylamine N-Oxide and the risk of stroke: A systematic review and dose-response meta-Analysis. *Nutrition Journal* 2020; 19: 76. doi:10.1186/s12937-020-00592-2

41. Missailidis C, Hallqvist J, Qureshi AR, et al. Serum trimethylamine-N-Oxide is strongly related to renal function and predicts outcome in chronic kidney disease. *PLoS One* 2016; 11(1): e0141738. doi:10.1371/journal.pone.0141738

42. Song R, Xu H, Dintica CS, et al. Associations Between Cardiovascular Risk, Structural Brain Changes, and Cognitive Decline. *J Am Coll Cardiol* 2020; 75(20): 2525-2534. doi:10.1016/j.jacc.2020.03.053

43. Dinu M, Abbate R, Gensini GF, Casini A, Sofi F. Vegetarian, vegan diets and multiple health outcomes: A systematic review with meta-analysis of observational studies. *Crit Rev Food Sci Nutr* 2017; 57(17) 3640-3649. doi:10.1080/10408398.2016.1138447

44. Heianza Y, Ma W, DiDonato JA, et al. Long-Term Changes in Gut Microbial Metabolite Trimethylamine N-Oxide and Coronary Heart Disease Risk. *J Am Coll Cardiol* 2020; 75(7): 763-772. doi:10.1016/j.jacc.2019.11.060

45. Yang JJ, Lipworth LP, Shu X-O, et al. Associations of choline-related nutrients with cardiometabolic and all-cause mortality: Results from 3 prospective cohort studies of blacks, whites, and Chinese. *Am J Clin Nutr* 2020; 111(3): 644-656. doi:10.1093/ajcn/nqz318

Chapter 11: Common health concerns about vegan and vegetarian diets

1. Global, Regional, and Country-Specific Lifetime Risks of Stroke, 1990 and 2016. *N Engl J Med* 2018. doi:10.1056/nejmoa1804492

2. O'Donnell MJ, et al. Global and regional effects of potentially modifiable risk factors associated with acute stroke in 32 countries (INTERSTROKE): a case-control study. *Lancet* 2016. doi:10.1016/S0140-6736(16)30506-2

3. Campbell T. A plant-based diet and stroke. *J Geriatric Cardiol* 2017. doi:10.11909/j.issn.1671-5411.2017.05.010

4. Feng Q, et al. Adherence to the dietary approaches to stop hypertension diet and risk of stroke: A meta-analysis of prospective studies. *Med (United States)* 2018. doi:10.1097/MD.0000000000012450

5. Saulle R, Lia L, De Giusti M, La Torre G. A systematic overview of the scientific literature on the association between Mediterranean Diet and the Stroke prevention. *Clin Ter* 2019. doi:10.7417/CT.2019.2166

6. Tong TYN, et al. Risks of ischaemic heart disease and stroke in meat eaters, fish eaters, and vegetarians over 18 years of follow-up: Results from the prospective EPIC-Oxford study. *Br Med J* 2019. doi:10.1136/bmj.l4897

7. Glenn AJ, et al. Relation of vegetarian dietary patterns with major cardiovascular outcomes: A systematic review and meta-analysis of prospective cohort studies. *Frontiers in Nutrition* 2019. doi:10.3389/fnut.2019.00080

8. Wang X, Dong Y, Qi X, Huang C, Hou L. Cholesterol levels and risk of hemorrhagic stroke: A systematic review and meta-analysis. *Stroke* 2013. doi:10.1161/STROKEAHA.113.001326

9. Chiu THT, et al. Vegetarian diet and incidence of total, ischemic, and hemorrhagic stroke in 2 cohorts in Taiwan. *Neurology* 2020. doi:10.1212/WNL.0000000000009093

10. Baden MY, et al. Quality of Plant-Based Diet and Risk of Total, Ischemic, and Hemorrhagic Stroke. *Neurology* 2021; 96(2021).

11. Chen GC, Lv DB, Pang Z, Liu QF. Red and processed meat consumption and risk of stroke: A meta-analysis of prospective cohort studies. *Eur J Clin Nutr* 2013. doi:10.1038/ejcn.2012.180

12. Melina V, Craig W, Levin S. Position of the Academy of Nutrition and Dietetics: Vegetarian Diets. *J Acad Nutr Diet* 2016. doi:10.1016/j.jand.2016.09.025

13. BDA. British Dietetic Association confirms well-planned vegan diets can support healthy living in people of all ages. (2017). Available at: www.bda.uk.com/resource/british-dietetic-association-confirms-well-planned-vegan-diets-can-support-healthy-living-in-people-of-all-ages.html.

14. Amit M, et al. Vegetarian diets in children and adolescents. *Paediatrics and Child Health* 2010. doi:10.1093/pch/15.5.303

References

15. Baroni L, et al. Vegan nutrition for mothers and children: Practical tools for healthcare providers. *Nutrients* 2019. doi:10.3390/nu11010005

16. Armstrong MK, et al. Association of Non–High-Density Lipoprotein Cholesterol Measured in Adolescence, Young Adulthood, and Mid-Adulthood With Coronary Artery Calcification Measured in Mid-Adulthood. *JAMA Cardiol* 2021. doi:10.1001/jamacardio.2020.7238

17. Palinski W, Napoli C. The fetal origins of atherosclerosis: maternal hypercholesterolemia, and cholesterol-lowering or antioxidant treatment during pregnancy influence in utero programming and postnatal susceptibility to atherogenesis. *FASEB J* 2002. doi:10.1096/fj.02-0226rev

18. Alberti G, et al. Type 2 diabetes in the Young: The Evolving Epidemic. The International Diabetes Federation Consensus Workshop. *Diabetes Care* 2004. doi:10.2337/diacare.27.7.1798

19. Sutter DO, Bender N. Nutrient status and growth in vegan children. *Nutr Res* 2021; 91: 13-25. doi.org/10.1016/j.nutres.2021.04.005

20. Weder S, Hoffmann M, Becker K, Alexy U, Keller M. Energy, macronutrient intake, and anthropometrics of vegetarian, vegan, and omnivorous children (1-3 years) in Germany (VeChi diet study). *Nutrients* 2019. doi:10.3390/nu11040832

21. Alexy U, et al. Nutrient intake and status of german children and adolescents consuming vegetarian, vegan or omnivore diets: Results of the vechi youth study. *Nutrients* 2021; 13.

22. Sanders TAB, Manning J. The growth and development of vegan children. *J Hum Nutr Diet* 1992. doi:10.1111/j.1365-277X.1992.tb00129.x

23. O'Connell JM, et al. Growth of vegetarian children: The Farm Study. *Pediatrics* 1989.

24. Schürmann S, Kersting M, Alexy U. Vegetarian diets in children: a systematic review. *Eur J Nutr* 2017. doi:10.1007/s00394-017-1416-0

25. Nathan I, Hackett AF, Kirby S. A longitudinal study of the growth of matched pairs of vegetarian and omnivorous children, aged 7-11 years, in the North-West of England. *Eur J Clin Nutr* 1997. doi:10.1038/sj.ejcn.1600354

26. Hebbelinck M, Clarys P, De Malsche A. Growth, development, and physical fitness of Flemish vegetarian children, adolescents, and young adults. *Am J Clin Nutr* 1999. doi:10.1093/ajcn/70.3.579s

27. Leung A, Otley A. Concerns for the use of soy-based formulas in infant nutrition. *Paediatr Child Health* 2009. doi:10.1093/pch/14.2.109

28. Health Canada, Canadian Paediatric Society, Dietitians of Canada & Breastfeeding Committee for Canada. Nutrition for healthy term infants: recommendations from birth to six months. *Can J Diet Pract Res* 2012. doi:10.3148/73.4.2012.204

29. British Dietetic Association. Paediatric group position statement on the use of soya protein for infants. *J Fam Health Care* 2003.

30. Vandenplas Y, et al. Safety of soya-based infant formulas in children. *Br J Nutr* 2014. doi:10.1017/S0007114513003942

31. Sinai T, et al. Consumption of soy-based infant formula is not associated with early onset of puberty. *Eur J Nutr* 2019. doi:10.1007/s00394-018-1668-3

32. Sinai T, et al. Infantile consumption of soy-based formula is not associated with early onset of puberty and overweight in school aged children. *Endocr Rev* 2016.

33. Foster M, Samman S. Vegetarian diets across the lifecycle: Impact on zinc intake and status. *Adv Food Nutr Res* 2015. doi:10.1016/bs.afnr.2014.11.003

34. Baines SK. Zinc and vegetarian diets. *Med J Aust* 2012. doi:10.5694/mjao11.11493

35. Gibson RS, Heath ALM, Szymlek-Gay EA. Is iron and zinc nutrition a concern for vegetarian infants and young children in industrialized countries? *Am J Clin Nutr* 2014. doi:10.3945/ajcn.113.071241

36. Pawlak R, Bell K. Iron Status of Vegetarian Children: A Review of Literature. *Ann Nutr Metabol* 2017. doi:10.1159/000466706

37. Hovinen T, et al. Vegan diet in young children remodels metabolism and challenges the statuses of essential nutrients. *EMBO Mol Med* 2021. doi:10.15252/emmm.202013492

38. Yen CE, Yen CH, Huang MC, Cheng CH, Huang YC. Dietary intake and nutritional status of vegetarian and omnivorous preschool children and their parents in Taiwan. *Nutr Res* 2008. doi:10.1016/j.nutres.2008.03.012

39. Farberov S. US vegan parents who eat only raw fruit and vegetables are charged with MURDER for the starvation death of their 18-month-old son who was found weighing only 17lbs. *Daily Mail* 19 December 2019. www.dailymail.co.uk/news/article-7810073/Vegan-parents-charged-murder-baby-sons-starvation-death.html (accessed 26 October 2021)

40. Gregory A. Vegan parents sentenced for allowing toddler to become so malnourished her bones fractured. *Independent* 22 August 2019. www.independent.co.uk/news/world/australasia/vegan-baby-malnourished-diet-australia-nsw-unvaccinated-bone-disease-rickets-a9074081.html

41. Cundiff DK, Harris W. Case report of 5 siblings: Malnutrition? Rickets? DiGeorge syndrome? Developmental delay? *Nutr J* 2006. doi:10.1186/1475-2891-5-1

42. Amoroso S, et al. Acute small bowel obstruction in a child with a strict raw vegan diet. *Arch Dis Child* 2019. doi:10.1136/archdischild-2018-314910

43. Lemoine A, Giabicani E, Lockhart V, Grimprel E, Tounian P. Case report of nutritional rickets in an infant following a vegan diet. *Arch Pediatr* 2020. doi:10.1016/j.arcped.2020.03.008

44. Lund AM. Questions about a vegan diet should be included in differential diagnostics of neurologically abnormal infants with failure to thrive. *Acta Paediatrica* 2019. doi:10.1111/apa.14805

45. Segovia-Siapco G, Burkholder-Cooley N, Tabrizi SH, Sabaté J. Beyond meat: A comparison of the dietary intakes of vegetarian and non-vegetarian adolescents. *Front Nutr* 2019. doi:10.3389/fnut.2019.00086

46. Segovia-Siapco G, et al. Animal protein intake is associated with general

adiposity in adolescents: The teen food and development study. *Nutrients* 2020. doi:10.3390/nu12010110

47. Perry CL, McGuire MT, Neumark-Sztainer D, Story M. Adolescent vegetarians: How well do their dietary patterns meet the healthy people 2010 objectives? *Arch Pediatr Adolesc Med* 2002. doi:10.1001/archpedi.156.5.431

48. Waldmann A, Koschizke JW, Leitzmann C, Hahn A. Dietary intakes and lifestyle factors of a vegan population in Germany: Results from the German vegan study. *Eur J Clin Nutr* 2003. doi:10.1038/sj.ejcn.1601629

49. Weikert C, et al. Vitamin and Mineral Status in a Vegan Diet. *Dtsch Aerzteblatt Online* 2020. doi:10.3238/arztebl.2020.0575

50. Melnik BC. Evidence for acne-promoting effects of milk and other insulinotropic dairy products. *Nestle Nutrition Workshop Series: Pediatric Program* 2011. doi:10.1159/000325580

51. Messina M, Rogero MM, Fisberg M, Waitzberg D. Health impact of childhood and adolescent soy consumption. *Nutr Rev* 2017. doi:10.1093/nutrit/nux016

52. Sabaté J, Wien M. Vegetarian diets and childhood obesity prevention. *Am J Clin Nutr* 2010. doi:10.3945/ajcn.2010.28701F

53. Rogers IS, et al. Diet throughout childhood and age at menarche in a contemporary cohort of British girls. *Public Health Nutr* 2010. doi:10.1017/S1368980010001461

54. Kissinger DG, Sanchez A. The association of dietary factors with the age of menarche. *Nutr Res* 1987. doi:10.1016/S0271-5317(87)80003-9

55. Jansen EC, Marín C, Mora-Plazas M, Villamor E. Higher childhood red meat intake frequency is associated with earlier age at menarche. *J Nutr* 2016. doi:10.3945/jn.115.226456

56. Wu Y, et al. Higher poultry consumption was associated with an earlier age at menarche. *Acta Paediatr* 2020. doi:10.1111/apa.15554

57. Villamor E, Jansen EC. Nutritional Determinants of the Timing of Puberty. *Ann Rev Public Health* 2016. doi:10.1146/annurev-publhealth-031914-122606

58. Hamajima N, et al. Menarche, menopause, and breast cancer risk: Individual participant meta-analysis, including 118 964 women with breast cancer from 117 epidemiological studies. *Lancet Oncol* 2012. doi:10.1016/S1470-2045(12)70425-4

59. Charalampopoulos D, McLoughlin A, Elks CE, Ong KK. Age at menarche and risks of all-cause and cardiovascular death: A systematic review and meta-analysis. *Am J Epidemiol* 2014. doi:10.1093/aje/kwu113

60. Cheng TS, Day FR, Lakshman R, Ong KK. Association of puberty timing with type 2 diabetes: A systematic review and meta analysis. *PLoS Med* 2020. doi:10.1371/JOURNAL.PMED.1003017

61. Maleki N, Kurth T, Field AE. Age at menarche and risk of developing migraine or non-migraine headaches by young adulthood: A prospective cohort study. *Cephalalgia* 2017. doi:10.1177/0333102416677999

62. Sioka C, et al. Age at menarche, age at menopause and duration of fertility as risk factors for osteoporosis. *Climacteric* 2010. doi:10.3109/13697130903075337

63. Cheng G, et al. Diet quality in childhood is prospectively associated with the timing of puberty but not with body composition at puberty onset. *J Nutr* 2010. doi:10.3945/jn.109.113365

64. Duan R, et al. The overall diet quality in childhood is prospectively associated with the timing of puberty. *Eur J Nutr* 2020. doi:10.1007/s00394-020-02425-8

65. Zuromski KL, Witte TK, Smith AR, et al. Increased prevalence of vegetarianism among women with eating pathology. *Eat Behav* 2015; 19: 24-27. doi: 10.1016/j.eatbeh.2015.06.017.

66. Robinson-O'Brien R, Perry CL, Wall MM, Story M, Neumark-Sztainer D. Adolescent and Young Adult Vegetarianism: Better Dietary Intake and Weight Outcomes but Increased Risk of Disordered Eating Behaviors. *J Am Diet Assoc* 2009; 109(4): 648-655. doi: 10.1016/j.jada.2008.12.014.

67. Sergentanis TN, Chelmi M-E, Liampas A, et al. Vegetarian Diets and Eating Disorders in Adolescents and Young Adults: A Systematic Review. *Children* 2020; 8(1): 12. doi: 10.3390/children8010012

68. Bardone-Cone AM, Fitzsimmons-Craft EE, Harney MB, et al. The Inter-Relationships between Vegetarianism and Eating Disorders among Females. *J Acad Nutr Diet* 2012; 112(8): 1247-1252. doi: 10.1016/j.jand.2012.05.007.

69. O'Connor MA, Touyz SW, Dunn SM, Beumont PJV. Vegetarianism in anorexia nervosa? A review of 116 consecutive cases. *Med J Aust* 1987; 147(11-12): 540-542. doi: 10.5694/j.1326-5377.1987.tb133677.x.

70. Heiss S, Coffino JA, Hormes JM. Eating and health behaviors in vegans compared to omnivores: Dispelling common myths. *Appetite* 2017; 118: 129-135. doi: 10.1016/j.appet.2017.08.001.

71. Melina V, Craig W, Levin S. Position of the Academy of Nutrition and Dietetics: Vegetarian Diets. *J Acad Nutr Diet* 2016. doi:10.1016/j.jand.2016.09.025

72. Sebastiani G, Barbero AH, Borras-Novell C, et al. The effects of vegetarian and vegan diet during pregnancy on the health of mothers and offspring. *Nutrients* 2019; 11(3). doi:10.3390/nu11030557

73. Perak AM, Lancki N, Kuang A, et al. Associations of Maternal Cardiovascular Health in Pregnancy With Offspring Cardiovascular Health in Early Adolescence. *JAMA* 2021; 325(7): 658-668. doi: 10.1001/jama.2021.0247

74. Hever J, Cronise RJ. Plant-based nutrition for healthcare professionals: Implementing diet as a primary modality in the prevention and treatment of chronic disease. *J Geriatr Cardiol* 2017. doi:10.11909/j.issn.1671-5411.2017.05.012

75. Volkert D, Beck AM, Cederholm T, et al. ESPEN guideline on clinical nutrition and hydration in geriatrics. *Clin Nutr* 2019; 38(1): 10-47.

References

doi:10.1016/j.clnu.2018.05.024

76. Katz DL, Doughty KN, Geagan K, Jenkins DA, Gardner CD. Perspective: The Public Health Case for Modernizing the Definition of Protein Quality. *Adv Nutr* 2019. doi:10.1093/advances/nmz023

77. Franceschi C, Garagnani P, Parini P, Giuliani C, Santoro A. Inflammaging: a new immune–metabolic viewpoint for age-related diseases. *Nature Rev Endocrinol* 2018. doi:10.1038/s41574-018-0059-4

78. Pan A, Sun Q, Bernstein AM, et al. Red meat consumption and mortality: Results from 2 prospective cohort studies. *Arch Intern Med* 2012; 172(7): 555-563. doi:10.1001/archinternmed.2011.2287

79. GBD 2019 Demographics Collaborators. Global age-sex-specific fertility, mortality, healthy life expectancy (HALE), and population estimates in 204 countries and territories, 1950–2019: a comprehensive demographic analysis for the Global Burden of Disease Study 2019. *Lancet* 2020; 396(10258): 1160-1203. doi:10.1016/S0140-6736(20)30977-6

80. Struijk EA, Hagan KA, Fung TT, et al. Diet quality and risk of frailty among older women in the Nurses' Health Study. *Am J Clin Nutr* 2020; 111(4): 877-883. doi:10.1093/ajcn/nqaa028

81. Ortolá R, Struijk EA, García-Esquinas E, Rodríguez-Artalejo F, Lopez-Garcia E. Changes in Dietary Intake of Animal and Vegetable Protein and Unhealthy Aging. *Am J Med* 2020. doi:10.1016/j.amjmed.2019.06.051

82. Foscolou A, Cunha NM, Naumovski N, et al. The association between whole grain products consumption and successful aging: A combined analysis of MEDIS and ATTICA epidemiological studies. *Nutrients* 2019; 11(6). doi:10.3390/nu11061221

83. Gil-Salcedo A, Dugravot A, Fayosse A, et al. Healthy behaviors at age 50 years and frailty at older ages in a 20-year follow-up of the UK Whitehall II cohort: A longitudinal study. *PLoS Med* 2020; 17(7): e1003147. doi:10.1371/journal.pmed.1003147

84. Willett WC, Ludwig DS. Milk and health. *N Eng J Med* 2020. doi:10.1056/NEJMra1903547

85. Brondani JE, Comim FV, Flores LM, Martini LA, Premaor MO. Fruit and vegetable intake and bones: A systematic review and meta-analysis. *PLoS One* 2019. doi:10.1371/journal.pone.0217223

86. Livingston G, et al. Dementia prevention, intervention, and care. *Lancet* 2017. doi:10.1016/S0140-6736(17)31363-6

87. Livingston G, et al. Dementia prevention, intervention, and care: 2020 report of the Lancet Commission. *Lancet* 2020. doi:10.1016/S0140-6736(20)30367-6

88. World Health Organization (WHO). *Risk reduction of cognitive decline and dementia: WHO guidelines*. WHO, Geneva; 5 February 2019. www.who.int/publications/i/item/risk-reduction-of-cognitive-decline-and-dementia (accessed 24 October 2021)

89. Barnard ND, et al. Dietary and lifestyle guidelines for the prevention of Alzheimer's disease. *Neurobiol Aging* 2014.

doi:10.1016/j.neurobiolaging.2014.03.033

90. Mao X, et al. Intake of vegetables and fruits through young adulthood is associated with better cognitive function in midlife in the US general population. J Nutr; 2019. doi:10.1093/jn/nxz076

91. Kowalski K, Mulak A. Brain-gut-microbiota axis in Alzheimer's disease. *J Neurogastroenterol Motil* 2019. doi:10.5056/jnm18087

92. Linus Pauling Institute. Flavonoids. Oregon State University; 2017. https://lpi.oregonstate.edu/mic/dietary-factors/phytochemicals/flavonoids (accessed 24 October 2021)

93. Shishtar E, Rogers GT, Blumberg JB, Au R, Jacques PF. Long-term dietary flavonoid intake and change in cognitive function in the Framingham Offspring cohort. *Public Health Nutr* 2020. doi:10.1017/S136898001900394X

94. Holland TM, Agarwal P, Wang Y, et al. Dietary flavonols and risk of Alzheimer dementia. *Neurology* 2020; 94(16): e1749-e1756. doi:10.1212/WNL.0000000000008981

95. Yuan C, Chen H, Wang Y, et al. Dietary carotenoids related to risk of incident Alzheimer dementia (AD) and brain AD neuropathology: a community-based cohort of older adults. *Am J Clin Nutr* 2020; 113(1): 200-208. doi: 10.1093/ajcn/nqaa303

96. Srisuwan P. Prevention of Dementia Through Modifiable Risk Factors. In: Farooqui T, Farooqui AA. *Diet and Exercise in Cognitive Function and Neurological Diseases.* John Wiley & Sons; 2015. doi:10.1002/9781118840634.ch15

97. Amen DG, Harris WS, Kidd PM, Meysami S, Raji CA. Quantitative Erythrocyte Omega-3 EPA Plus DHA Levels are Related to Higher Regional Cerebral Blood Flow on Brain SPECT. *J Alzheim Dis* 2017. doi:10.3233/JAD-170281

98. Zhang Y, et al. Intakes of fish and polyunsaturated fatty acids and mild-to-severe cognitive impairment risks: A dose-response meta-analysis of 21 cohort studies. *Am J Clin Nutr* 2016. doi:10.3945/ajcn.115.124081

99. Bakre AT, et al. Association between fish consumption and risk of dementia: A new study from China and a systematic literature review and meta-analysis. *Public Health Nutrition* 2018. doi:10.1017/S136898001800037X

100. Dangour AD, Andreeva VA, Sydenham E, Uauy R. Omega 3 fatty acids and cognitive health in older people. *Br J Nutr* 2012. doi:10.1017/S0007114512001547

101. Dobersek U, et al. Meat and mental health: a systematic review of meat abstention and depression, anxiety, and related phenomena. *Critical Rev Food Sci Nutr* 2021. doi:10.1080/10408398.2020.1741505

102. Lundh A, Lexchin J, Mintzes B, Schroll JB, Bero L. Industry sponsorship and research outcome. *Cochrane Database Syst Rev* 2017. doi:10.1002/14651858.MR000033.pub3

103. Coggen D, Rose G, Barker DJP. Chapter 8. Case-control and cross

sectional studies. In: Epidemiology for the Uninitiated. BMJ; 1997.

104. Gómez-Donoso C, et al. Ultra-processed food consumption and the incidence of depression in a Mediterranean cohort: the SUN Project. *Eur J Nutr* 2020. doi:10.1007/s00394-019-01970-1

105. Li Y, Lv M-R, Wei Y-J, et al. Dietary patterns and depression risk: A meta-analysis. *Psychiatry Research* 2017; 253: 373-382. doi:10.1016/j.psychres.2017.04.020

106. O'Neil A, Berk M, Itsiopoulos C, et al. A randomised, controlled trial of a dietary intervention for adults with major depression (the 'SMILES' trial): Study protocol. *BMC Psychiatry* 2013; 13: 114. doi:10.1186/1471-244X-13-114

107. Parletta N, Zarnowiecki D, Cho J, et al. A Mediterranean-style dietary intervention supplemented with fish oil improves diet quality and mental health in people with depression: A randomized controlled trial (HELFIMED). *Nutr Neurosci* 2019; 22(7): 474-487. doi:10.1080/1028415X.2017.1411320

108. Agarwal U, Mishra S, Xu J, et al. A multicenter randomized controlled trial of a nutrition intervention program in a multiethnic adult population in the corporate setting reduces depression and anxiety and improves quality of life: the GEICO study. *Am J Health Promot* 2015; 29(4): 245-254. doi:10.4278/ajhp.130218-QUAN-72

109. Adjibade M, Lemogne C, Touvier M, et al. The inflammatory potential of the diet is directly associated with incident depressive symptoms among French adults. *J Nutr* 2019; 149(7): 1198-1207. doi:10.1093/jn/nxz045

110. Medawar E, Huhn S, Villringer A, Witte AV. The effects of plant-based diets on the body and the brain: a systematic review. *Translational Psychiatry* 2019; 9: 226. doi:10.1038/s41398-019-0552-0

111. Li F, Liu X, Zhang D. Fish consumption and risk of depression: A meta-analysis. *J Epidemiol Community Health* 2015. doi:10.1136/jech-2015-206278

112. D'Ascenzo F, et al. Atherosclerotic coronary plaque regression and the risk of adverse cardiovascular events: A meta-regression of randomized clinical trials. *Atherosclerosis* 2013. doi:10.1016/j.atherosclerosis.2012.10.065

113. Daida H, Dohi T, Fukushima Y, Ohmura H, Miyauchi K. The goal of achieving atherosclerotic plaque regression with lipid-lowering therapy: Insights from IVUS trials. *J Atheroscler Thromb* 2019; 26(7): 592-600. doi: 10.5551/jat.48603.

114. Ornish D, Brown SE, Scherwitz JH, et al. Can lifestyle changes reverse coronary heart disease?. The Lifestyle Heart Trial. *Lancet* 1990; 336(8708): 129-133. doi:10.1016/0140-6736(90)91656-U

115. Esselstyn CB, Gendy G, Doyle J, Golubic M, Roizen MF. A way to reverse CAD? *J Fam Pract* 2014. doi:10.1109/APUSNCURSINRSM.2017.8072476

116. Appleby PN, Key TJ. The long-term health of vegetarians and vegans. in *Proceedings of the Nutrition Society* 2016. doi:10.1017/S0029665115004334

117. Dinu M, Abbate R, Gensini GF, Casini A, Sofi F. Vegetarian, vegan diets

and multiple health outcomes: A systematic review with meta-analysis of observational studies. *Crit Rev Food Sci Nutr* 2017. doi:10.1080/10408398.2016.1138447

118. Kane-Diallo A, Srour B, Sellem L, et al. Association between a pro plant-based dietary score and cancer risk in the prospective NutriNet-santé cohort. *Int J Cancer* 2018; 143(9): 2168-2176. doi:10.1002/ijc.31593

119. Kim H, Caulfield LE, Garcia-Larsen V, et al. Plant-based diets and incident CKD and kidney function. *Clin J Am Soc Nephrol* 2019; 14(5): 682-691. doi:10.2215/CJN.12391018

120. Appleby PN, Crowe FL, Bradbury KE, Travis RC, Key TJ. Mortality in vegetarians and comparable nonvegetarians in the United Kingdom. *Am J Clin Nutr* 2016; 103(1): 218-230. doi:10.3945/ajcn.115.119461

121. Kim H, Caulfield LE, Rebholz CM. Healthy plant-based diets are associated with lower risk of all-cause mortality in US Adults. *J Nutr* 2018; 148(4): 624-631. doi:10.1093/jn/nxy019

122. Kim H, Caulfield LE, Garcia-Larsen V, et al. Plant-Based Diets Are Associated With a Lower Risk of Incident Cardiovascular Disease, Cardiovascular Disease Mortality, and All-Cause Mortality in a General Population of Middle-Aged Adults. *J Am Heart Assoc* 2019; 8(16): e012865. doi:10.1161/JAHA.119.012865

123. Gardner CD, Trepanowski JF, del Gobbo LC. Effect of low-fat VS low-carbohydrate diet on 12-month weight loss in overweight adults and the association with genotype pattern or insulin secretion the DIETFITS randomized clinical trial. *JAMA* 2018; 319(7): 667-679. doi:10.1001/jama.2018.0245

124. Asnicar F, Berry SE, Valdes AN, et al. Microbiome connections with host metabolism and habitual diet from 1,098 deeply phenotyped individuals. *Nat Med* 2021; 27(2): 321-322. doi:10.1038/s41591-020-01183-8

Chapter 12: Additional benefits of a plant-based diet

1. Williams R, Alexander G, Armstrong I, et al. Disease burden and costs from excess alcohol consumption, obesity, and viral hepatitis: fourth report of the Lancet Standing Commission on Liver Disease in the UK. *Lancet* 2018; 391(10125): 1097-1107. doi:10.1016/S0140-6736(17)32866-0

2. Abenavoli L, di Renzo L, Boccuto L, et al. Health benefits of Mediterranean diet in nonalcoholic fatty liver disease. *Expert Rev Gastroenterol Hepatol* 2018; 12(9): 873-881. doi: 10.1080/17474124.2018.1503947.

3. Mazidi M, Kengne A. Higher adherence to plant-based diets are associated with lower likelihood of fatty liver. *Clin Nutr* 2018; 38(4): 1672-1677. doi: 10.1016/j.clnu.2018.08.010.

References

4. Chiu TH, Lin MN, Pan WH, Chen YC, Lin CL. Vegetarian diet, food substitution, and nonalcoholic fatty liver. *Tzu Chi Med J* 2018; 30(2): 102-109. doi: 10.4103/tcmj.tcmj_109_17.

5. Chiarioni G, Popa SL, Dalbeni A, et al. Vegan Diet Advice Might Benefit Liver Enzymes in Nonalcoholic Fatty Liver Disease: an Open Observational Pilot Study. *J Gastrointestin Liver Dis* 2021; 30(1): 81-87. doi: 10.15403/jgld-3064.

6. Kahleova H, Petersen KF, Shulman GI, Shulman GI. Effect of a Low-Fat Vegan Diet on Body Weight, Insulin Sensitivity, Postprandial Metabolism, and Intramyocellular and Hepatocellular Lipid Levels in Overweight Adults. *JAMA Netw Open* 2020; 3(11): e2025454. doi: 10.1001/jamanetworkopen.2020.25454.

7. Turney BW, Appleby PN, Reynard JM, et al. Diet and risk of kidney stones in the Oxford cohort of the European Prospective Investigation into Cancer and Nutrition (EPIC). *Eur J Epidemiol* 2014; 29(5): 363-369. doi: 10.1007/s10654-014-9904-5.

8. Ferraro PM, Bargagli M, Trinchieri A, Gambaro G. Risk of kidney stones: Influence of dietary factors, dietary patterns, and vegetarian–vegan diets. *Nutrients* 2020; 12(3): 779. doi: 10.3390/nu12030779.

9. Chen Y-C, Chang CC, Chiu THT, Lin M-N, Lin C-L. The risk of urinary tract infection in vegetarians and non-vegetarians: a prospective study. *Sci Rep* 2020; 10(1): 906. doi: 10.1038/s41598-020-58006-6.

10. Jakobsen L, Spangholm DJ, Pedersen K, et al. Broiler chickens, broiler chicken meat, pigs and pork as sources of ExPEC related virulence genes and resistance in Escherichia coli isolates from community-dwelling humans and UTI patients. *Int J Food Microbiol* 2010; 142(1-2): 264-272. doi: 10.1016/j.ijfoodmicro.2010.06.025.

11. Clinton CM, O'Brien S, Law J, Renier CM, Wendt MR. Whole-Foods, Plant-Based Diet Alleviates the Symptoms of Osteoarthritis. *Arthritis* 2015; 2015: 798152. doi: 10.1155/2015/708152.

12. Aleksandrova K, Koelman L, Rodrigues CE. Dietary patterns and biomarkers of oxidative stress and inflammation: A systematic review of observational and intervention studies. *Redox Biol* 2021. doi:10.1016/j.redox.2021.101869

13. Chiu THT, Liu CH, Chang CC, Lin MN, Lin CL. Vegetarian diet and risk of gout in two separate prospective cohort studies. *Clin Nutr* 2020; 39(3): 837-844. doi: 10.1016/j.clnu.2019.03.016

14. Barnard ND, Scialli AR, Hurlock D, Bertron P. Diet and sex-hormone binding globulin, dysmenorrhea, and premenstrual symptoms. *Obstet Gynecol* 2000. doi:10.1016/S0029-7844(99)00525-6

15. Barnard ND, Kahleova H, Holtz DN, et al. The Women's Study for the Alleviation of Vasomotor Symptoms (WAVS): a randomized, controlled trial of a plant-based diet and whole soybeans for postmenopausal women. *Menopause* 2021; 28(10): 1150-1156. doi: 10.1097/GME.0000000000001812

16.   Chen MN, Lin CC, Liu CF. Efficacy of phytoestrogens for menopausal symptoms: A meta-analysis and systematic review. *Climacteric* 2015; 18.

17.   Daily JW, Ko B-S, Ryuk J, et al. Equol Decreases Hot Flashes in Postmenopausal Women: A Systematic Review and Meta-Analysis of Randomized Clinical Trials. *J Med Food* 2019; 22(2): 127-139. doi: 10.1089/jmf.2018.4265

18.   Tomova A, Bukovsky I, Rembert E, et al. The Effects of Vegetarian and Vegan Diets on Gut Microbiota. *Front Nutr* 2019; 6:47. doi: 10.3389/fnut.2019.00047

19.   Sekikawa A, Higashiyama A, Lopresti BJ, et al. Associations of equol-producing status with white matter lesion and amyloid-β deposition in cognitively normal elderly Japanese. *Alzheimer's Dement* 2020; 6(1): e12089. doi: 10.1002/trc2.12089.

20.   Haghighatdoost F, Bellissimo N, Totosy De Zepetnek JO, Rouhani MH. Association of vegetarian diet with inflammatory biomarkers: A systematic review and meta-analysis of observational studies. Public Health Nutrition 2017. doi:10.1017/S1368980017001768

21.   Carlsen MH, Halvorsen BL, Holte K, et al. The total antioxidant content of more than 3100 foods, beverages, spices, herbs and supplements used worldwide. *Nutr J* 2010; 9: 3. doi:10.1186/1475-2891-9-3

22.   Chiba M, Nakane K, Komatsu M. Westernized Diet is the Most Ubiquitous Environmental Factor in Inflammatory Bowel Disease. *Perm J* 2019; 23.

23.   Alwarith J, Kahleova H, Rembert E, et al. Nutrition Interventions in Rheumatoid Arthritis: The Potential Use of Plant-Based Diets. A Review. *Front Nutr* 2019; 6: 141. doi: 10.3389/fnut.2019.00141.

24.   Lewandowska M, Dunbar K, Kassam S. Managing Psoriatic Arthritis With a Whole Food Plant-Based Diet: A Case Study. *Am J Lifestyle Med* 2021. doi:10.1177/1559827621993435

25.   Sandefur K, Kahleova H, Desmond AN, Elfrink E, Barnard ND. Crohn's disease remission with a plant-based diet: A case report. *Nutrients* 2019; 11.

26.   Goldner B. Six Week Raw Vegan Nutrition Protocol Rapidly Reverses Lupus Nephritis: A Case Series. *Int J Dis Reversal Prev* 2019; 1(1). doi.org/10.22230/ijdrp.2019v1n1a47

27.   Chiba M, Tsuji T, Nakane K, et al. Induction with Infliximab and a Plant-Based Diet as First-Line (IPF) Therapy for Crohn Disease: A Single-Group Trial. *Perm J* 2017; 21: 17-009. doi: 10.7812/TPP/17-009.

28.   Westermann R, Zobbe K, Cordtz R, Haugaard JH, Dreyer L. Increased cancer risk in patients with cutaneous lupus erythematosus and systemic lupus erythematosus compared with the general population: A Danish nationwide cohort study. *Lupus* 2021; 30.

29.   Luo X, Deng C, Fei Y, et al. Malignancy development risk in psoriatic arthritis patients undergoing treatment: A systematic review and meta-analysis. *Semin Arthritis Rheum* 2019; 48(4): 626-631.

References

doi: 10.1016/j.semarthrit.2018.05.009.

30. Ramage-Morin PL, Gilmour H. Prevalence of migraine in the canadian household population. *Health Reports* 2014; 25.

31. Global Burden of Desease Study 2013 Collaborators. Global, regional, and national incidence, prevalence, and years lived with disability for 301 acute and chronic diseases and injuries in 188 countries, 1990-2013: A systematic analysis for the Global Burden of Disease Study 2013. *Lancet* 2015; 386(9995): 743-800. doi.org/10.1016/S0140-6736(15)60692-4

32. Puledda F, Shields K. Non-pharmacological approaches for migraine. *Neurotherapeutics* 2018; 15(2): 336-345. doi: 10.1007/s13311-018-0623-6.

33. Bic Z, Blix GG, Hopp HP, Leslie FM, Schell MJ. The influence of a low-fat diet on incidence and severity of migraine headaches. *J Women's Health Gend-Based Med* 1999; 8(5): 623-630. doi: 10.1089/jwh.1.1999.8.623.

34. Bunner AE, Agarwal U, Gonzales JF, Valente F, Barnard N. D. Nutrition intervention for migraine: a randomized crossover trial. *J Headache Pain* 2014; 15(1): 69. doi: 10.1186/1129-2377-15-69

35. Chiu THT, Chang CC, Lin CL, Lin MN. A Vegetarian Diet Is Associated with a Lower Risk of Cataract, Particularly Among Individuals with Overweight: A Prospective Study. *J Acad Nutr Diet* 2020. doi:10.1016/j.jand.2020.11.003

36. Appleby PN, Allen NE, Key TJ. Diet, vegetarianism, and cataract risk. *Am J Clin Nutr* 2011; 93(5): 1128-1135. doi: 10.3945/ajcn.110.004028

37. Zampatti S, Ricci F, Cusumango A, et al. Review of nutrient actions on age-related macular degeneration. *Nutr Res* 2014; 34(2): 95-105. doi: 10.1016/j.nutres.2013.10.011.

38. Chakravarthy U, Wong TY, Fletcher A, et al. Clinical risk factors for age-related macular degeneration: A systematic review and meta-analysis. *BMC Ophthalmol* 2010; 10: 31. doi: 10.1186/1471-2415-10-31.

39. García-Layana A, Cabrera-López F, García-Arumí J, Arias-Barquet L, Ruiz-Moreno JM. Early and intermediate age-related macular degeneration: Update and clinical review. *Clin Interv Aging* 2017; 12: 1579-1587. doi: 10.2147/CIA.S142685.

40. Tsai CJ, Leitzmann MF, Willett WC, Giovannucci EL. Heme and non-heme iron consumption and risk of gallstone disease in men. *Am J Clin Nutr* 2007; 85.

41. Tsai CJ, Leitzmann MF, Willett WC, Giovannucci EL. Long-term intake of trans-fatty acids and risk of gallstone disease in men. *Arch Intern Med* 2005; 165.

42. Tsai CJ, Leitzmann MF, Willett WC, Giovannucci EL. Long-chain saturated fatty acids consumption and risk of gallstone disease among men. *Ann Surg* 2008; 247.

43. Wirth J, Joshi AD, Song M, et al. A healthy lifestyle pattern and the risk of symptomatic gallstone disease: Results from 2 prospective cohort studies. *Am J Clin Nutr* 2020; 112(3): 586-594. doi: 10.1093/ajcn/nqaa154.

44. Chen YC, Chiou C, Lin MN, Lin CL. The prevalence and risk factors for

gallstone disease in taiwanese vegetarians. *PLoS One* 2014; 9.

45. Chang CM, Chiu THT, Chang CC, Lin MN, Lin CL. Plant-based diet, cholesterol, and risk of gallstone disease: A prospective study. *Nutrients* 2019; 11.

46. Wirth J, Song M, Fung TT, et al. Diet-quality scores and the risk of symptomatic gallstone disease: A prospective cohort study of male US health professionals. *Int J Epidemiol* 2018; 47(6): 1938-1946. doi: 10.1093/ije/dyy210.

47. McConnell TJ, Appleby PN, Key TJ. Vegetarian diet as a risk factor for symptomatic gallstone disease. *Eur J Clin Nutr* 2017; 71.

48. Lin CL, Wang JH, Lin MN, Chang CC, Chiu THT. Vegetarian diets and medical expenditure in taiwan—a matched cohort study. *Nutrients* 2019. doi:10.3390/nu11112688

49. Cooper, J. Healthcare expenditure, UK Health Accounts: 2018. Office for National Statistics, UK. 28 April 2020. www.ons.gov.uk/peoplepopulationandcommunity/healthandsocialcare/healthcaresystem/bulletins/ukhealthaccounts/2018 (accessed 24 October 2021)

50. Statistics Canada. Three-fifths of total federal, provincial, territorial and local spending went to social protection, health care and education in 2019. 27 November 2020.

51. Canadian Institute for Health Information. National Health Expenditure Trends , 1975 to 2019. Canadian Institute for Health Information Report (2019). www150.statcan.gc.ca/n1/daily-quotidien/201127/dq201127a-eng.htm (accessed 24 October 2021)

52. Statista. Number of coronavirus (COVID-19) cases worldwide as of September 22, 2021, by country. (2021). www.statista.com/statistics/1043366/novel-coronavirus-2019ncov-cases-worldwide-by-country/ (accessed 3 October 2021)

53. Williamson EJ, Walker AJ, Bhaskaran K, et al. Factors associated with COVID-19-related death using OpenSAFELY. *Nature* 2020; 584(7821): 430-436. doi: 10.1038/s41586-020-2521-4

54. O'Hearn M, Liu J, Cudhea F, Micha R, Mozaffarian D. Coronavirus disease 2019 hospitalizations attributable to cardiometabolic conditions in the united states: A comparative risk assessment analysis. *J Am Heart Assoc* 2021; 10.

55. Calder PC. Nutrition, immunity and COVID-19. *BMJ Nutr Prev Health* 2020; 3(1): 74-92. doi: 10.1136/bmjnph-2020-000085.

56. Zheng D, Liwinski T, Elinav E. Interaction between microbiota and immunity in health and disease. *Cell Research* 2020; 30(6): 492-506. doi: 10.1038/s41422-020-0332-7.

57. Yeoh YK, Zuo T, Lui GC-Y, et al. Gut microbiota composition reflects disease severity and dysfunctional immune responses in patients with COVID-19. *Gut* 2021; 70(4): 698-706. doi: 10.1136/gutjnl-2020-323020.

58. McDonald D, Hyde E, Debelius JW, et al. American Gut: an Open

Platform for Citizen Science Microbiome Research. *mSystems* 2018; 3(3): e00031-18. doi:10.1128/msystems.00031-18

59. Kim H, Rebholz CM, Hegde S, et al. Plant-based diets, pescatarian diets and COVID-19 severity: A population-based case-control study in six countries. *BMJ Nutr Prev Health* 2021; 4: e000272. doi:10.1136/bmjnph-2021-000272

60. Merino J, Joshi AD, Nguyen LH, et al. Diet quality and risk and severity of COVID-19: a prospective cohort study. *Gut* 2021; 70(11): 2096-2104. doi:10.1136/gutjnl-2021-325353

61. Lopez-Leon S, Wegman-Ostrosky T, Perelman C, et al. More than 50 long-term effects of COVID-19: a systematic review and meta-analysis. *Sci Rep* 2021; 11. doi: 10.1101/2021.01.27.21250617

62. Storz MA. Lifestyle Adjustments in Long-COVID Management: Potential Benefits of Plant-Based Diets. *Curr Nutr Rep* 2021. doi:10.1007/s13668-021-00369-x

Chapter 13: Considerations for planetary health

1. Poore J, Nemecek T. Reducing food's environmental impacts through producers and consumers. *Science* 2018; 80. doi:10.1126/science.aaq0216

2. IPCC. Climate Change 2021: The Physical Science Basis. (2021). www.ipcc.ch/report/sixth-assessment-report-working-group-i/.

3. United Nations Convention on Climate Change. *Paris Agreement. 21st Conference of the Parties* (2015). doi:FCCC/CP/2015/L.9

4. Clark MA, et al. Global food system emissions could preclude achieving the 1.5° and 2°C climate change targets. *Science* 2020; 80. doi:10.1126/science.aba7357

5. Theurl MC, et al. Food systems in a zero-deforestation world: Dietary change is more important than intensification for climate targets in 2050. *Sci Total Environ* 2020. doi:10.1016/j.scitotenv.2020.139353

6. Sandström V, et al. The role of trade in the greenhouse gas footprints of EU diets. *Glob Food Sec* 2018. doi:10.1016/j.gfs.2018.08.007

7. Crippa, M. et al. Food systems are responsible for a third of global anthropogenic GHG emissions. *Nat Food* 2021; 2.

8. Rao S. Animal Agriculture is the Leading Cause of Climate Change - A position Paper. *J Ecol Soc* 2021; 32–33.

9. Saunois M, et al. The global methane budget 2000-2017. *Earth Syst Sci Data* 2020. doi:10.5194/essd-12-1561-2020

10. Hayek MN, Miller SM. Underestimates of methane from intensively raised animals could undermine goals of sustainable development. *Environmental Research Letters* 2021; 16.

11. United Nations Environment Programme. *Global Methane Assessment: Benefits and Costs of Mitigating Methane Emissions.* 2021.

12. Uwizeye A, et al. Nitrogen emissions along global livestock supply chains. *Nat Food* 2020. doi:10.1038/s43016-020-0113-y

13. Strokal M, et al. Alarming nutrient pollution of Chinese rivers as a result of agricultural transitions. *Environ Res Lett* 2016. doi:10.1088/1748-9326/11/2/024014

14. Berendes DM, Yang PJ, Lai A, Hu D, Brown J. Estimation of global recoverable human and animal faecal biomass. *Nat Sustain* 2018. doi:10.1038/s41893-018-0167-0

15. Borlee F, et al. Air pollution from livestock farms is associated with airway obstruction in neighboring residents. *Am J Respir Crit Care Med* 2017. doi:10.1164/rccm.201701-0021OC

16. Bourdrel T, Bind MA, Béjot Y, Morel O, Argacha JF. Cardiovascular effects of air pollution. *Archives of Cardiovascular Diseases* 2017. doi:10.1016/j.acvd.2017.05.003

17. Domingo NGG, et al. Air quality-related health damages of food. *Proc Natl Acad Sci USA* 2021; 118.

18. Eat Forum. *Diets for a Better Future*. 2020.

19. Hayek MN, Harwatt H, Ripple WJ, Mueller ND. The carbon opportunity cost of animal-sourced food production on land. *Nat. Sustain* 2021. doi:10.1038/s41893-020-00603-4

20. González-Sánchez EJ, et al. Conservation Agriculture and its contribution to the achievement of agri-environmental and economic challenges in Europe. *AIMS Agriculture and Food* 2016; 1.

21. Springmann M, et al. Health and nutritional aspects of sustainable diet strategies and their association with environmental impacts: a global modelling analysis with country-level detail. *Lancet Planet Heal* 2018. doi:10.1016/S2542-5196(18)30206-7

22. Bongaarts, J. IPBES, 2019. Summary for policymakers of the global assessment report on biodiversity and ecosystem services of the Intergovernmental Science-Policy Platform on Biodiversity and Ecosystem Services. *Popul Dev Rev* 2019; 45.

23. Ceballos G, Ehrlich PR, Raven PH. Vertebrates on the brink as indicators of biological annihilation and the sixth mass extinction. *Proc Natl Acad Sci* 2020.

24. WWF. Living Planet Report - 2018: Aiming higher. *Environmental Conservation* 2018; 26.

25. Bergstrom DM, et al. Combating ecosystem collapse from the tropics to the Antarctic. *Glob Chang Biol* 2021; 27.

26. Benton T, Bieg C, Harwatt H, Pudassaini R, Wellesley L. Food system impacts on biodiversity loss Three levers for food. Energy, Environment and Resources Programme (2021).

27. Garnett T, et al. Grazed and confused? Ruminating on Cattle, Grazing Systems, Methane, Nitrous Oxide, the Soil Carbon Sequestration Question-and what it All Means for Greenhouse Gas Emissions. *Food Clim Res Netw* 2017.

28. Hayek MN, Garrett RD. Nationwide shift to grass-fed beef requires larger

References

cattle population. *Environ Res Lett* 2018. doi:10.1088/1748-9326/aad401

29. Pieper M, Michalke A, Gaugler T. Calculation of external climate costs for food highlights inadequate pricing of animal products. *Nat Commun* 2020. doi:10.1038/s41467-020-19474-6

30. Willett W, et al. Food in the Anthropocene: the EAT–Lancet Commission on healthy diets from sustainable food systems. *Lancet*2019; 6736: 3–49.

31. Filazzola A, et al. The effects of livestock grazing on biodiversity are multi-trophic: a meta-analysis. *Ecology Letters* 2020. doi:10.1111/ele.13527

32. Bradbury RB, et al. The economic consequences of conserving or restoring sites for nature. *Nat Sustain* 2021. doi:10.1038/s41893-021-00692-9

33. DeLong C, Cruse R, Wiener J. The soil degradation paradox: Compromising our resources when we need them the most. *Sustainability (Switzerland)* 2015; 7.

34. Karlen DL, Rice CW. Soil degradation: Will humankind ever learn? *Sustainability (Switzerland)* 2015; 7.

35. Bertrand M, et al. Earthworm services for cropping systems. A review. *Agronomy for Sustainable Development* 2015; 35.

36. Kassam A, Friedrich T, Derpsch R. Global spread of Conservation Agriculture. *Int J Environ Stud* 2019; 76.

37. Kassam A. Advances in Conservation Agriculture, Volume 2: Practices and Benefits. *J Chem Inf Model* 2020; 53.

38. Rethinking Food and Agriculture. Rethinking Food and Agriculture (2021). doi:10.1016/c2017-0-04570-6

39. Kritee K, et al. High nitrous oxide fluxes from rice indicate the need to manage water for both long- and short-term climate impacts. *Proc Natl Acad Sci USA* 2018. doi:10.1073/pnas.1809276115

40. Stoop WA. The scientific case for system of rice intensification and its relevance for sustainable crop intensification. *Int J Agric Sustain* 2011. doi:10.1080/14735903.2011.583483

41. Thakur AK, Uphoff NT. How the system of rice intensification can contribute to climate-smart agriculture. *Agronomy Journal* 2017. doi:10.2134/agronj2016.03.0162

42. Uphoff NT. System of Rice Intensification. Responses to Frequently Asked Questions. (2015).

43. World Water Assessment Programme (WWAP). The United Nations World Water Development Report 2015: Water for a Sustainable World, Facts and Figures. *UN Water Rep* 2015.

44. Proveg. Plant Milk Report. (2019).

45. Food and Agriculture Organization of the United Nations. *The State of World Fisheries and Aquaculture 2016. Contributing to food securtiy and nutrition for all.* Rome, 2016. doi:92-5-105177-1 www.fao.org/3/i5555e/i5555e.pdf

46. Kumar BR. et al. A state of the art review on the cultivation of algae for energy and other valuable products: Application, challenges, and opportunities. *Renewable and Sustainable Energy Reviews* 2021; 138.

47. Thomas K, Obaidullah F, Dorey DC. Ghost Gear : the Abandoned Fishing Nets Haunting. *Greenpeace Ger* 2019.

48. Lebreton L, et al. Evidence that the Great Pacific Garbage Patch is rapidly accumulating plastic. *Sci Rep* 2018; 8.

49. Barboza LGA, et al. Microplastics in wild fish from North East Atlantic Ocean and its potential for causing neurotoxic effects, lipid oxidative damage, and human health risks associated with ingestion exposure. *Sci Total Environ* 2020; 717.

50. Wang W, Ge J, Yu, X. Bioavailability and toxicity of microplastics to fish species: A review. *Ecotoxicol Environ Saf* 2020; 189.

51. Development Initiatives. *2020 Global Nutrition Report: Action on equity to end malnutrition.* https://globalnutritionreport.org/reports/2020-global-nutrition-report/ (accessed 24 October 2021)

52. Berners-Lee M, Kennelly C, Watson R, Hewitt CN. Current global food production is sufficient to meet human nutritional needs in 2050 provided there is radical societal adaptation. *Elementa* 2018; 6.

53. Hickel J. The true extent of global poverty and hunger: questioning the good news narrative of the Millennium Development Goals. *Third World Q* 2016; 37.

54. Ritchie H, Roser M. Meat and Dairy Production. *Our World Data* 2019.

55. Chen C, Chaudhary A, Mathys A. Nutritional and environmental losses embedded in global food waste. *Resour Conserv Recycl* 2020; 160.

56. EU Committee. Counting the Cost of Food Waste: EU Food Waste Prevention. *Auth House Lords* 2014. doi:10.1111/j.1365-313X.2010.04415.x

57. Pais DF, Marques AC, Fuinhas JA. Reducing Meat Consumption to Mitigate Climate Change and Promote Health: but Is It Good for the Economy? *Environ Model Assess* 2020; 25.

58. Shepon A, Eshel G, Noor E, Milo R. The opportunity cost of animal based diets exceeds all food losses. *Proc Natl Acad Sci USA* 2018; 115.

59. Pedro G de AV, et al. Determinants of the Brazilian Amazon deforestation. *African J Agric Res* 2017; 12.

60. Tyukavina A, et al. Types and rates of forest disturbance in Brazilian Legal Amazon, 2000–2013. *Sci Adv* 2017; 3.

61. EK. et al. Outbreaks of Shiga Toxin-Producing Escherichia coli Linked to Sprouted Seeds, Salad, and Leafy Greens: A Systematic Review. *J Food Prot* 2019.

62. Abebe E, Gugsa G, Ahmed M. Review on Major Food-Borne Zoonotic Bacterial Pathogens. *J Trop Med* 2020; 2020.

63. Kirk MD, et al. World Health Organization Estimates of the Global and Regional Disease Burden of 22 Foodborne Bacterial, Protozoal, and Viral Diseases, 2010: A Data Synthesis. *PLoS Med* 2015. doi:10.1371/journal.pmed.1001921

64. European Food Safety Authority (EFSA). *Salmonella the most common cause of foodborne outbreaks in the European Union.* 12 December 2019.

References

www.ecdc.europa.eu/en/news-events/salmonella-most-common-cause-foodborne-outbreaks-european-union (accessed 24 October 2021)

65. Canadian Food Inspection Agency. Causes of food poisoning. Gov. Canada (2012). https://inspection.canada.ca/food-safety-for-consumers/fact-sheets/food-poisoning/eng/1331151916451/1331152055552 (accessed 24 October 2021)

66. Landers TF, Cohen B, Wittum TE, Larson EL. A review of antibiotic use in food animals: Perspective, policy, and potential. *Public Health Reports* 2012. doi:10.1177/003335491212700103

67. Courtenay M, et al. Tackling antimicrobial resistance 2019–2024 – The UK's five-year national action plan. *J Hosp Infec* 2019. doi:10.1016/j.jhin.2019.02.019

68. Caruso GG. Antibiotic resistance in Escherichia coli from farm livestock and related analytical methods: A review. *J AOAC International* 2018. doi:10.5740/jaoacint.17-0445

69. Van Gompel L, et al. Description and determinants of the faecal resistome and microbiome of farmers and slaughterhouse workers: A metagenome-wide cross-sectional study. *Environ Int* 2020. doi:10.1016/j.envint.2020.105939

70. Manyi-Loh C, Mamphweli S, Meyer E, Okoh A. Antibiotic use in agriculture and its consequential resistance in environmental sources: Potential public health implications. *Molecules* 2018; 23(4): 795. doi:10.3390/molecules23040795

71. Losasso C, Cesare di A, Mastrorilli E, et al. Assessing antimicrobial resistance gene load in vegan, vegetarian and omnivore human gut microbiota. *Int J Antimicrob Agents* 2018; 52: 702–705. doi: 10.1016/j.ijantimicag.2018.07.023

72. Milanović V, Osimani A, Aquilanti L, et al. Occurrence of antibiotic resistance genes in the fecal DNA of healthy omnivores, ovo-lacto vegetarians and vegans. *Mol Nutr Food Res* 2017; 61(9). doi: 10.1002/mnfr.201601098

73. Milanović V, Aquilanti L, Tavoletti S, et al. Distribution of antibiotic resistance genes in the saliva of healthy omnivores, ovo-lacto-vegetarians, and vegans. *Genes* 2020; 11(9): 1088. doi.org/10.3390/genes11091088

74. Van Boeckel TP, Glennon EE, Chen D, et al. Reducing antimicrobial use in food animals. *Science* 2017; 357(6358): 1350-1352. doi: 10.1126/science.aao1495.

75. Andersen KG, Rambaut A, Lipkin WI, Holmes EC, Garry RF. The proximal origin of SARS-CoV-2. *Nature Medicine* 2020; 26: 450-452. doi:10.1038/s41591-020-0820-9

76. Morse SS, Mazet JAK, Woolhouse M, et al. Prediction and prevention of the next pandemic zoonosis. *Lancet* 2012; 380(9857): 1956-1965. doi:10.1016/S0140-6736(12)61684-5

77. Gibb R, Redding DW, Chin KQ, et al. Zoonotic host diversity increases in human-dominated ecosystems. *Nature* 2020; 584: 398-402.

doi.org/10.1038/s41586-020-2562-8

78. Peters A. Covid-19 shows the need for a global animal law. *Derecho Anim* 2020; 11(4): 86-97. doi: 105565/rev/da.150

79. Rossi J, Garner SA. Industrial Farm Animal Production: A Comprehensive Moral Critique. *J Agric Environ Ethics* 2014; 27: 479-522. doi.org/10.1007/s10806-014-9497-8

80. Espinosa R, Tago D, Treich N. Infectious Diseases and Meat Production. *Environ Resour Econ* 2020; 76: 1-26. doi: 10.1007/s10640-020-00484-3

81. USDA-NASS. United States Department of Agriculture, National Agricultural Statistics Service. 2017 Census of Agriculture. 2017 Census of Agriculture (2019).
www.nass.usda.gov/Publications/AgCensus/2017/index.php

82. Tanner WD, Toth DJA, Gundlapalli AV. The pandemic potential of avian influenza A(H7N9) virus: A review. Epidemiology and Infection 2015; 143(16): 3359-3374. doi: 10.1017/S0950268815001570

83. Nuñez IA, Ross TM. A review of H5Nx avian influenza viruses. *Ther Adv Vaccines Immunother* 2019; 7: 1-15. doi: 10.1177/2515135518821625

84. Voronina OL, Ryzhova NN, Aksenova E, et al. Genetic features of highly pathogenic avian influenza viruses A(H5N8), isolated from the European part of the Russian Federation. *Infect Genet Evol* 2018; 63: 144-150. doi: 10.1016/j.meegid.2018.05.022

Chapter 14: Final thoughts

1. Abbafati C et al. Global burden of 87 risk factors in 204 countries and territories, 1990–2019: a systematic analysis for the Global Burden of Disease Study 2019. *Lancet* 2020; 396.

2. Woolf SH, Schoomaker H. Life Expectancy and Mortality Rates in the United States, 1959-2017. *JAMA* 2019; 322.

3. Parry L, Steel N, Ford J. Slowing of life expectancy in the UK: Global Burden of Disease Study 2016. *Lancet* 2018; 392.

4. Bittner V. The New 2019 AHA/ACC Guideline on the Primary Prevention of Cardiovascular Disease. *Circulation* 2020. doi:10.1161/CIRCULATIONAHA.119.040625

5. Rock CL, et al. American Cancer Society guideline for diet and physical activity for cancer prevention. *Cancer J Clin* 2020. doi:10.3322/caac.21591

6. Kelly J, Karlsen M, Steinke G. Type 2 Diabetes Remission and Lifestyle Medicine: A Position Statement From the American College of Lifestyle Medicine. *Am J Lifestyle Med* 2020; 14.

7. GBD Diet Collaborators. Health effects of dietary risks in 195 countries, 1990–2017: a systematic analysis for the Global Burden of Disease Study 2017. *Lancet* 2019.

References

8.   Abbasi J. Medical students around the world poorly trained in nutrition. *JAMA* 2019; 322.

9.   Crowley J, Ball L, Hiddink GJ. Nutrition in medical education: a systematic review. *Lancet Planet Heal* 2019. doi:10.1016/S2542-5196(19)30171-8

10.   Bodai B. Lifestyle Medicine: A Brief Review of Its Dramatic Impact on Health and Survival. *Perm J* 2017. doi:10.7812/TPP/17-025

11.   American College of Lifestyle Medicine. What is lifestyle medicine? https://lifestylemedicine.org/What-is-Lifestyle-Medicine (2021).

12.   Kassam S, Dehghan L, Freeman L. How to help patients transition to a healthy and sustainable plant-based diet. *Br J Gen Practice* 2021; 71.

Index

Index

Index

Index

IGF-1 (insulin-like growth factor 1), 8, 38, 41–42, 47, 56, 58, 92, 153
iliac arteries, **219**
immune system and COVID-19, 182–183
  see also autoimmune disease
individualised (personalised) diets, 167–168
indole-3-carbinol, 87–88
industrialisation (agriculture), 45, 103, 203
  animal farming, 204–205
  see also food-industry-sponsored / funded studies
infants and babies
  peanut allergy, 126
  soya formulas, 149
infections
  foodborne, 65, 172, 202–203
  urinary tract, 171–172
  zoonoses, 202, 204–205, **222**
  see also antibiotics; pandemics
inflammation
  in arthritis, 172
  chronic, 41, 163
influenza, avian (bird flu), 205
insulin, 167
  administration, 82
  resistance, 15, 22, 41, 80–81, 82, 104, 108, 123, 169, 170, **219–220**
insulin-like growth factor (IGF-1), 8, 38, 41–42, 47, 56, 58, 92, 153
Intergovernmental Panel on Climate Change (IPCC), 187
International Agency for Research on Cancer (IARC), 84
international dietary guidelines, 25–26, 208
INTERSTROKE study, 145
Inuit and fish, 74
iodine, 140
  dairy and, 55–56
  pregnancy and, 156
iron, 33–34, 211
  deficiency, 33
    children, 59–60, 149–150
    red meat and, 33–34
irritable bowel syndrome, 98, 117–118
ischaemia, **220**

ischaemic heart disease *see* heart disease
ischaemic stroke, 145, 146–147, 147
isoflavones, 115, 117, 128, 174, **220**
  see also flavonoids

Jenkins, Dr David, 20, 108
juices (fruit and vegetables), 22
  fasting and juicing, 91–94
  store-bought, 93

ketogenic diet, 103, 104, 105
Keys, Ancel, 30
kidney
  potassium and diabetes and problems with, 82–83
  stones, 171

lactase, 10, 35, 52
lactic acid bacteria and fermented milk products dairy, 60
lacto-ovo vegetarianism, 5, 53
lactose, 10, 35
  intolerance, 10, 52
lacto-vegetarianism, 5
Lancet Commission on Dementia, 158
land use change, 191
  from animal farming to growing crops, 200–201
lauric acid, 29, 134, 135
LDL cholesterol, **218, 220**
  adolescents, and atherosclerosis in later life, 148
  coconut oil and, 134–135
  stroke and, 146
leaky gut, 22, 110
lectins, 110–111, 139
legumes *see* beans and legumes
lens cataracts, 177
lifestyle factors (impacting on health and well-being), 11
  COVID-19, 181
  dementia, 158
  IGF-1 and, 56
lifestyle medicine, 208–209
  hierarchies of evidence applied to (HEALM), 9
  see also American College of Lifestyle Medicine

Index

Index

Also from Hammersmith Health Books...

Feeding Your Vegan Child

A practical guide to plant-based nutrition

By Sandra Hood

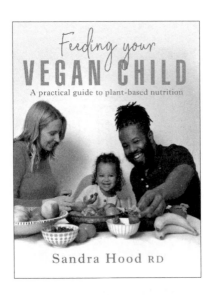

Whether you are vegan and planning a pregnancy or a health professional needing further information on nutritional guidelines for a vegan infant, this is an essential practical guide by a specialist NHS dietitian with many years of clinical experience. It takes you through all nutritional aspects of pregnancy up to early childhood and on to the teenage years following a purely plant-based diet.

Also from Hammersmith Health Books...

Living PCOS Free

How to regain your hormonal health and go from surviving to thriving with Polycystic Ovary Syndrome

By Dr Nitu Bajekal and Rohini Bajekal

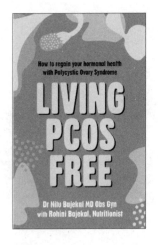

This practical guide will show you how to identify and successfully manage this common but under-diagnosed condition using proven lifestyle approaches alongside western medicine. With over 35 years of clinical experience, Dr Nitu Bajekal, AKA 'the 'Plant-Based Gynae,' and Nutritionist Rohini Bajekal, break through misinformation, providing clarity and support to help you tackle your symptoms - from irregular periods to acne and anxiety.